Your Baby Can Self-Feed, Too

ALSO BY GILL RAPLEY, coauthored with TRACEY MURKETT

Baby-Led Weaning: *The Essential Guide—How to Introduce Solid Foods and Help Your Baby Grow Up a Happy and Confident Eater*

The Baby-Led Weaning Cookbook: *Delicious Recipes That Will Help Your Baby Learn to Eat Solid Foods—and That the Whole Family Will Enjoy*

The Baby-Led Weaning Cookbook—Volume 2: *99 More No-Stress Recipes for the Whole Family*

Baby-Led Breastfeeding: *Follow Your Baby's Instincts for Relaxed and Easy Nursing*

Your Baby Can Self-Feed, Too

ADAPTED BABY-LED WEANING
for Children with Developmental Delays or Other Feeding Challenges

Jill Rabin, MS

Gill Rapley, PhD

THE EXPERIMENT

NEW YORK

The Experiment, LLC
220 East 23rd Street, Suite 600
New York, NY 10010-4658
theexperimentpublishing.com

The Experiment's books are available at special discounts when purchased in bulk for premiums and sales promotions as well as for fund-raising or educational use. For details, contact us at info@theexperimentpublishing.com.

Library of Congress Cataloging-in-Publication Data available upon request

ISBN 978-1-61519-902-0
Ebook ISBN 978-1-61519-903-7

Cover and text design by Beth Bugler
Cover photograph by Chereesca Bejasa

Manufactured in the United States of America

First printing September 2022
10 9 8 7 6 5 4 3 2 1

CONTENTS

PREFACE BY JILL RABIN

The first time I heard a lecture by Gill Rapley, pioneer of baby-led weaning (BLW), I was immediately transfixed. A colleague, Gail Macklin, had loaned me a DVD about the BLW approach and I became mesmerized by the footage of babies as young as 6 months feeding themselves with the same foods that their families were eating. When I saw how BLW worked for neurotypical babies, I knew I had to figure out a way to help babies with motor challenges learn to eat in the same way. What I didn't know was that this DVD would change the path of my career as a feeding therapist forever.

My work is primarily with neurodiverse babies with a range of diagnoses, including Down syndrome and Noonan syndrome, as well as babies born prematurely and those with a feeding aversion. I wanted to develop a way that these babies could learn to eat solid foods in the same self-directed way as their peers. Initially, I focused on babies with Down syndrome, many of whom were being spoon fed by adults into their second year of life, while continuing to drink from bottles rather than straws and cups and doing minimal self-feeding. Over the course of a few years, I discovered that it is not only possible for these babies to feed themselves but that there are huge benefits for them, too. Using observation, and a process of trial and error (and always with the full involvement of the baby's parents), I devised and refined the approach that I now call *adapted baby-led weaning* (ABLW).

I began by developing ways to help babies with motor challenges—such as limited muscular strength and difficulty with refined hand and finger movements—feed themselves using different food shapes and textures. I also experimented with bridge devices, such as silicone feeders and pre-loaded spoons, as I found the babies often struggled initially when relying on their hands and fingers. I was so excited to see how using these devices, with gentle and responsive support for the hand-to-mouth action, was helping them self-feed and learn to chew.

I found Gill's contact information on her website and decided, albeit apprehensively, to email her about my adapted approach. I knew, from her book *Baby-Led Weaning: The Essential Guide*, that she and her coauthor Tracey Murkett were unsure whether BLW was appropriate for babies with developmental challenges but theorized that it had the potential to be therapeutic. I wanted to show her just how well her ideas *do* work with this population. However, while I was convinced that adapting BLW was good for my patients, I worried that Gill would not approve of the use of feeding devices and other adaptations, since they are not part of the core concept of BLW. I felt strongly that these activities could act as a bridge, enabling babies facing feeding challenges to transition much more quickly to self-feeding than was generally assumed to be possible.

I reached out to Gill in July 2014, outlining how I had adapted her methods for neurodiverse babies and asking whether she would like to see some of the videos I had made of the babies I was seeing (with their parents' permission). I waited with trepidation for her response for what seemed like an eternity (but was in fact one week—she had been on vacation). I could hardly believe it when she said she was very interested in what I was doing and eager to learn more! From this initial contact, a friendship evolved between the two of us "BLW nerds," who share a passion for the approach. We exchanged current information and research on BLW, as well as videos and photos of babies self-feeding. We also discussed how best to describe and promote my adapted approach, how to educate colleagues, and how to respond to those who made disparaging remarks. With Gill's encouragement I started to speak more widely about my work to groups of professionals and parents, but in the back of my mind I knew I wanted to reach a wider audience.

My first lecture on ABLW was in 2016, at a conference for feeding therapists in Illinois. My methods were initially met with disdain and skepticism and I was told by therapist friends in the audience that some of the attendees thought what I was doing was outrageous, and potentially dangerous. They felt that babies with feeding challenges needed to be spoon fed by an adult and that spoon feeding was a necessary step in feeding development. I knew this wasn't the case but I wasn't sure how to convince others. I kept plugging away at my practice, seeing every day the benefits of ABLW but feeling frustrated that no one else was able to witness firsthand how beneficial— and safe—this approach was.

The big breakthrough came in the summer of 2018, when I met Lori Overland, a speech-language pathologist, at a weeklong orofacial myology course in New Jersey. Lori is well known in the pediatric feeding world and is a popular lecturer and author of books about feeding. She and I bonded over our feeding work with the 0-to-3-year-old population, and babies with Down syndrome in particular. Over lunch every day, we would sit together and discuss our different feeding cases. I eventually got up the nerve to show her some videos of my neurodiverse patients feeding themselves. She would later tell me that she initially thought what I was doing was ill-advised, as it seemed to her that some of the babies were using compensatory patterns to eat with this approach. Nevertheless, when she returned home she started trying bridge devices with a few of her patients. She quickly saw the benefits when ABLW was combined with the sensory-motor approach she had devised (described in chapter 8) and asked me if I would be willing to combine our approaches. She suggested we submit a proposal to the American Speech and Hearing Association (ASHA) for a joint presentation to our peers at the ASHA national convention, one of the largest gatherings of feeding professionals in the country. Our vision became a reality in 2019, when we showcased the "Sensory-Motor Approach to Baby-Led Weaning" in Orlando, Florida.

Lori's reputation meant that many of her colleagues, also accomplished in the field of feeding, attended our presentation. Her endorsement of, and belief in, ABLW brought the idea to the forefront of the specialty, which meant it could no longer be ignored. That day marked a shift in many people's perception of what might be possible, and interest in the approach started to gain speed. The following year Lori and I were invited to write a guest post for the online blog *Pediatric Feeding News*. In parallel, 2020 saw the launch of the Instagram account @ableappetites, which Sara Quirk and Sabrina Smiley Evans, both moms of babies with Down syndrome, had developed specifically to help families of babies with this diagnosis transition to solids using family foods. At the time of writing, a plethora of websites and social media accounts are embedding the concept of BLW and finger foods as first foods into our culture.[1] A baby-led approach for *all* babies is here to stay.

After twelve years of implementing ABLW with many different babies, my techniques and methods have become more refined, systematic, and effective. Today, I combine them with Lori's sensory-motor approach to create strong foundational feeding skills and facilitate self-feeding for the babies I see in my practice. The results are just amazing!

Fast forward to today and I'm thrilled to partner with Gill in writing this book. It's a distillation of everything we've learned—and it's for you, whether you're a parent or a professional. Gill and I believe that, with the right support from medical and feeding professionals and tailored guidance for their parents, babies with feeding challenges can learn to feed themselves and become independent, intuitive, and adventurous eaters just like their typically developing peers. We fervently hope that in the not-too-distant future, BLW and ABLW will be seen as a viable alternative to a reliance on spoon feeding and purees for all babies. It really does have the potential to change lives.

I'd like to dedicate this book to the two people who have been instrumental in getting me to this point. My former boss and mentor Perrie Kominsky launched my career into the feeding world. She was a forward-thinking, lifelong learner and my biggest cheerleader. She would be so proud. And then there's my friend and colleague Gail Macklin, who handed me that DVD back in 2010. Gail, it is because of you that I ventured into the BLW realm, and as a result my life and the lives of so many little ones with feeding challenges have been forever positively changed.

INTRODUCTION

Baby-led weaning (BLW) is an approach to the introduction of solid foods in which the baby shares family meals and feeds herself pieces of food with her hands rather than being spoon fed with purees. It's fast becoming *the* way to introduce solid foods for typically developing babies. But what if your baby's development is atypical, or if she has specific medical or other feeding challenges? Then this book is for you! It explains how BLW can be adapted to work for all babies, maximizing their abilities in relation to feeding while also supporting their wider development.

It's never too early to start thinking about how your baby will navigate the move toward independent eating and sharing family foods. It's also not too late if you've already started down that road and have a few questions. Either way, we think you will find this book helpful. We recommend that you share the information in it with the therapists who are supporting you, so that you can work together toward the same goals for your baby.

Babies are capable of far more than they are often given credit for, but it's easy for their abilities and desires to be overridden—especially if they face challenges that other babies don't. Too often, babies who have feeding difficulties end up having feeding done *to* them rather than being supported to play an active part in nourishing themselves. A baby-led approach allows all babies to achieve their potential in relation to eating, whatever the obstacles they—and their parents—face.

Baby-led weaning is about sharing meals with your baby, trusting her abilities, following her lead, facilitating self-feeding, and supporting her to manage foods of different shapes, sizes, textures, and consistency. It's about learning and skill development and responding to her appetite, not about getting food into her. She may need to start a little later, progress more slowly than her peers, or take a slightly different route, but once she has developed the skills she needs to get food to her mouth and chew it, she'll be able to follow the regular baby-led weaning approach that so many families are now discovering.

Ideally, you and your baby will be supported in your journey by an experienced medical, developmental, and feeding team that can help her first to establish a strong gross motor base and foundational feeding skills, and then to progress to more complex skills, via an appropriate pre-feeding program (see page 126) and therapeutic feeding plan (see page 129). While you may be constrained by the available providers in your area, it's worth seeking out professionals who truly understand the value of a baby-led approach so that you can work together to achieve the best outcomes for your child. Each baby is unique.

Whichever way you choose to tackle the introduction of solid foods, your child's progress won't exactly mirror that of any other baby. So, deciding to let her show you what she can do, and what help she needs (if any) at every step of the way, is a great mindset to adopt. You will not only be helping her learn to eat a large variety of different foods but also be supporting the development of a healthy relationship with food and a love for shared mealtimes.

A note to professionals

As baby-led weaning has continued to receive ever wider exposure, increasing numbers of parents of babies whose development follows a typical path are eagerly implementing it, with great results. Meanwhile, the body of research that supports it is growing rapidly. However, adapting the approach for use with babies who face challenges has not generally been seen as a realistic proposition. Pioneering work by a small number of practitioners is showing that adapted BLW is not only feasible but has unexpected and far-reaching benefits for this population.

As a health professional with a special interest in infant feeding, you may have been hesitant about recommending BLW because of fears about how the baby who has feeding challenges will cope with handling, chewing, and swallowing table foods. In much of our training—especially those of us who are feeding therapists—we have been taught that it is up to us to control the feeding in order to keep babies safe. We have also been persuaded that purees are a necessary first step in transitioning to solid foods. It can be hard to let go of what appear to be such fundamental principles. For this reason, many health professionals discourage families whose babies struggle with feeding from attempting BLW, fearing that it will prove impossible, or even dangerous. Unfortunately, this means that parents who wish to implement it are forced to get their information from sources such as social media, leaving them vulnerable to misinformation and suggestions that are inappropriate for their baby.

It is our belief that ABLW can benefit all babies whose progress with feeding may not follow the typical pattern, and that their parents would welcome the expert guidance of a feeding professional intimately familiar with the support for skill development and the selection of food texture, shape, and size that are crucial to this approach. Our intention in writing this book is therefore not to criticize your existing knowledge but rather to encourage you to reassess it and apply it in different ways. Adapted BLW is based primarily on principles you already know or intuit, rather than on new knowledge, whether that be the operation of the gag reflex or the importance of enabling babies to act autonomously. Your background in child development—especially oral motor development and feeding—will guide you in selecting safe food shapes and textures based on the baby's skill level; what may feel different is the trust you invest in the baby.

Adapted baby-led weaning is an exciting addition to the bag of tricks that professionals rely on to help babies and children become safe, independent, and adventurous self-feeders. It is our hope that this book will equip, empower, and inspire you to implement this approach with your clients, and that you and their parents will be as thrilled with the results as we are.

What you will find in this book

There are nine chapters in this book. The early chapters provide some background and explain the challenges that babies whose development follows an atypical path can face when learning to eat; the later ones deal with the practicalities of implementing ABLW. There is a logic to how we've laid them out, but you can start at whatever point makes the most sense to you.

Chapter 1 is a brief history of how spoon feeding and pureed baby food came to be seen as the "normal" way to introduce solids and what has happened in recent years to challenge that assumption. Chapter 2 describes the approach known as baby-led weaning: what it is, how it works, and the benefits that an adapted version offers for babies with feeding challenges. Chapter 3 explains how babies learn to eat, focusing not just on chewing skills but also on the part played by reflexes, sensory learning, dexterity, and gross motor development.

Chapter 4 outlines which babies are at special risk for feeding challenges, whether that's because of inborn factors or because of circumstances that arise in their first few months. Chapter 5 looks at how to plan ahead to ensure the best outcomes from ABLW, from sourcing the right professional support and building a solid foundation of sensory experience and motor skills, through devising a pre-feeding program and therapeutic feeding plan, to recognizing when the baby is truly ready to start. Chapter 6 deals with the practical issues of implementing ABLW at home: choosing a high chair, preparing for mess, planning family mealtimes, and helping to make your baby's eating experiences focused and positive.

Chapter 7 is all about preparing food in ways that will help your baby to become an independent eater. It looks at issues of shape, size, and texture and how these features contribute to the development of new skills while consolidating existing ones. Chapter 8 describes the therapeutic process that will support your baby's learning, starting with the importance of engaging his interest and gaining his permission so that he feels in control of what is happening. It also describes the bridge devices and therapeutic techniques that are key features of ABLW and explores what an individual baby's progress might look like. Finally, chapter 9 deals with some common concerns of parents and caregivers about topics that include throwing food, gagging, slow progress, and how to switch from spoon feeding to ABLW.

In between the chapters you will find nine real-life stories. These are babies that Jill has worked with, and we are immensely grateful to their parents for their willingness to share their experiences. It so happens that, in each case, it's the baby's mother who has attended the majority of the consultations, but this should not be taken to mean that his or her other parent hasn't been very much involved. It's also important to note that all these babies are individuals and the therapeutic techniques described have been tailored to their particular oral motor, feeding, and nutritional needs. They should not be assumed to be appropriate in all cases, no matter how similar the situation may appear.

This book is intended primarily for parents and feeding therapists, but we anticipate that it will be of value to anyone interested in the feeding of babies and young children, especially those who face feeding challenges. On a practical level, we hope it will serve as a guide to anyone actively supporting an individual baby's move from milk feeding to family meals, helping them to navigate the ups and downs of the transition in a way that empowers everyone involved. We are fully respectful of the many different parenting possibilities that exist, and of the preferences of individuals in how they describe themselves and their situation. However, for clarity, we have opted to use the term *human milk* to indicate milk produced by human breast tissue, and *breastfeeding* to refer to the action of feeding directly from the parent's body. For simplicity, we have referred to the parent producing this milk as the mother, using the pronoun "she." In order to be fair to all babies, we've alternated "he" and "she" by chapter.

> The yearning to nourish our babies and for them to be included from the outset does not change regardless of their delays, disabilities, or number of chromosomes.
>
> Sara Quirk and Sabrina Smiley Evans, @ableappetites

1

....

How We Got Here

In the developed Western world, when we think of introducing solid food to babies, the picture that comes to mind is of a caregiver bringing spoonfuls of puree to a baby's mouth. It seems that this is how things were always done. Often, these images are associated with cherished childhood memories and long-established family traditions. However, spoon feeding and purees are a relatively recent phenomenon with—we are increasingly discovering—no basis in how most babies develop. As we will see, these practices mostly originated in situations where mothers were not able or available to breastfeed and were then perpetuated by the developing culture.

In recent times, research has shown that babies do not need anything other than human milk or infant formula until they are 6 months old, by which time they are developing skills that allow them to feed themselves and to manage a variety of textures. However, the idea of purees has been so ingrained in our understanding of feeding babies that we assume they are essential. We have lost the genuine human tradition of introducing babies to solid foods according to their biological needs and skills. These methods allowed babies to eat independently, to develop jaw strength and fine motor skills, to achieve optimal development of the upper airways, to swallow efficiently and safely, and to respond to their bodies' senses of hunger and satiation. All babies deserve the chance to discover how to feed themselves and to have an enjoyable relationship with food—including babies whose development follows a path that is different from their peers'. To help them achieve this we need to untangle ourselves from conventional wisdom and prevailing customs and realign to practices that are grounded in basic biology and infant development.

A brief history of baby food

In prehistoric times, breastfeeding was the only available option for a newborn, and the only way to ensure his survival. With breastfeeding going well, and in the absence of childcare manuals or healthcare practitioners to advise them otherwise, parents would have had no reason to introduce solid foods until their child showed an interest in sampling the foods they themselves were eating. The beginning of the move away from human milk, also known as weaning, was thus inevitably *baby-led*.

Fossil evidence indicates that babies typically began chewing real foods from around 6 months.[1] Given that the first teeth required for chewing—molars—do not erupt in humans until between 13 and 19 months, and the second molars not until the child's third year, the period between the first solid foods and the last breastfeed would almost certainly have stretched well into toddlerhood, with milk providing an extended nutritional bridge as the infant adapted to a mixed diet.[2] It seems likely, too, that during this time caregivers would have pre-chewed tough, fibrous foods, such as meats and root vegetables, to assist the baby's digestion.[3] This is the evolutionary model for what is now referred to as *complementary feeding*. The idea of giving purees to babies appears to have originated not as a means of introducing solid foods but as a substitute for breastfeeding. From the sixteenth until the eighteenth century, babies who were failing to thrive, or for whom human milk was not available, were fed "pap" (flour or bread crumbs cooked in water or milk with water) or "panada" (cereal or bread cooked in broth)—either on its own or with animal milk. Feeding involved the use of a "papboat" (see photo 50), from which the food could be poured or blown into the baby's mouth.[4] Back then, the first solid foods were not given until babies were much older, so they graduated to table food, not purees. In the nineteenth century, cow's milk began to be routinely adapted for young babies—by the addition of other ingredients—and the use of pap and panada declined.

In the first half of the twentieth century, the expanding influence of doctors over birth, childcare, and infant feeding began to replace the natural sharing of information within families and the passing on of child-rearing knowledge from mother to daughter. As a result, practices were introduced— such as the routine separation of mothers and babies and the imposition of rigid feeding schedules—that led to a decline in breastfeeding. At the same time, the shortcomings of the available substitutes for human milk were becoming apparent. An alternative approach to the problem of babies not thriving on human milk was to introduce home-prepared versions of familiar family foods, to be given alongside the milk feeds. Doctors saw no harm in prescribing these "solid" foods for very young babies, with the result that, in the space of a generation, foods that had previously not been introduced until 7 months or later were being given as early as 6 weeks. Kitchen blenders weren't yet in common use, so the preparation of homemade foods for babies was time-consuming and tedious. In addition, more and more mothers were working outside the home, meaning that they had even less time for laborious household tasks. Commercial companies quickly stepped in to solve the problem by producing "strained" foods, originally in metal cans and later in glass jars.

The first branded baby foods appeared in the US in the 1920s and their use expanded rapidly, chiefly through endorsement by doctors and the impact of aggressive advertising. Advertisements directed at the general public preyed on the vulnerability of mothers, leading them to believe that commercial baby foods were better, safer, and more nutritious than those made at home—in relation to vitamin levels, for example. Some messages were even geared toward fathers, telling them how these new foods would make life easier for their wives![5] The babies themselves made their own unknowing contribution: The use of preservatives and flavor enhancers to ensure a long shelf life gave the products a distinctive flavor that babies quickly learned to prefer to home-cooked food. By the 1940s, jarred baby foods were well and truly embedded in North American culture. (For further reading on the growth of the baby food industry, see page 262.)

In spite of a recent return to the later introduction of solid foods and home-cooked meals for infants, the baby food market is still strong and influential. Since the 1960s many companies have responded to the demand for organically produced foods, while others have created a supposed need for snack foods for babies. The belief that prolonged use of purees is inevitable for babies and children who face feeding challenges may well be an additional contributing factor. According to the Zion Market Research company, "the global baby food market accounted for USD 72.01 billion in 2020 and is expected to reach USD 109.7 billion by 2028," representing a compound annual growth rate of 6.2 percent.[6]

The phenomenon of spoon feeding

Spoons have existed for many thousands of years, yet their role in the routine feeding of babies is a relatively recent phenomenon, cemented by the revolution in infant feeding that took place in the first half of the twentieth century. The perceived need to give solid foods to ever younger babies, coupled with strict rules about how much and when, as well as the emergence of commercial foods, meant that spoon feeding rapidly became synonymous with babyhood. Pureed baby foods and spoon feeding by a caregiver are intertwined. The rationale goes like this: The only way to get food into a baby who is too immature to pick it up for himself is for a caregiver to actively put it into his mouth; since the baby is also too young to chew, the food must be pureed; the most convenient tool for picking up and delivering a puree is a spoon; and since the baby cannot yet use a spoon independently, he must be fed by a caregiver. What is surprising is that this circular logic persists even though we now know that most babies do not need solid food until they are old enough to get it to their mouth themselves (using their hands) and to chew it, making both purees and spoon feeding by a caregiver unnecessary. There is an accompanying assumption that the first solid foods have to be *semi*solid (that is, pureed) in consistency—irrespective of the age or skill level of the baby—because they represent a transition from one type of feeding to another. And yet there is no evidence that such a transition requires the use of foods that are themselves transitional in nature,[7] either in their content (mixed with human milk) or in their texture (pureed), *unless* the transition is being imposed before the baby is developmentally ready to negotiate it.

The lingering belief that babies must be spoon fed in the early weeks of complementary feeding is common among both parents and professionals, including many pediatricians and therapists. Most textbooks about infant feeding mention spoon feeding when describing the transition from milk feedings to solid foods. Some even suggest that this represents the developmental norm, and that babies will not learn to bring their lips together to make the bilabial sounds *muh, buh,* and *puh* unless they are spoon fed. Thus, a typical feeding-skills checklist will identify the ability to take food from a spoon as a key milestone that should normally precede biting and chewing, with no acknowledgment that spoon feeding of infants is a relatively modern phenomenon, unknown in many cultures. The feeding progression outlined in these same texts commonly calls for gradually increasing thickness and the inclusion of small lumps in the presented food. Foods that require biting and chewing are often not recommended until 9 months or later—and then only as finger foods to be offered alongside those fed by spoon. Similarly, discussions of self-feeding tend to relate to the baby's feeding himself with a spoon rather than using his hands. The idea that a spoon isn't any more necessary than a fork until the child is able to use it independently is, to many people, quite strange.

From spoons to other gadgets

Marketing of baby products isn't limited to food; parents are inundated with advertisements for numerous feeding devices that are promoted as must-haves. These range from bottles to bowls, and bibs to blenders. Although these items are often presented as being beneficial for babies, in reality most of them exist for the convenience of parents. Of course, this in itself isn't a bad thing—parenting is time-consuming and hard work. The problem comes when the device gets in the way of the baby's developing important skills. Two examples of gadgets that can have a negative impact on babies' progress with feeding are sippy cups and pouches. The way a baby uses his mouth affects how his oral cavity grows. There is evidence that prolonged sucking on an artificial nipple or pacifier can cause the palate to develop a high arch, which may be accompanied by narrowing of the airway and can potentially lead to snoring, sleep apnea, overcrowding of teeth, and difficulties with speech.[8] Sippy cups can encourage an immature pattern of tongue-thrusting and suckling that has the potential to exacerbate these problems, while spill-proof, spoutless 360 cups promote over-activation of the upper lip and overuse of the jaw, as the baby works to extract the liquid from the cup.[9]

According to the manufacturers, food pouches are intended to be emptied into a bowl and the contents fed to the baby by spoon. In practice, however, they are often given to babies and toddlers to hold, with the aim that they will extract the food by sucking and squeezing. This bypasses the opportunity for the baby to develop complex oral skills. Because no chewing is required, swallowing tends to be rapid, so eating this way can lead to excessive food intake. It can also make the baby less willing to chew more complex foods. Additionally, pouches separate eating from the social environment of a shared meal and the sensory experience of real food; sucking applesauce from a pouch is a long way from the experience of biting into an apple. Both pouches and no-spill cups encourage parents to allow their toddler to carry the device with them, sucking intermittently over long periods of time. This encourages on-off eating (grazing), which can interfere with the baby's awareness of feelings of hunger and satiety. It can also mean that the teeth are in prolonged contact with sugary foods and drinks, leading to tooth decay and possibly even impacting the growth of the bones of the mouth and face.

Not all gadgets are bad (although they all have the potential to be misused). As we will see (chapter 8), some have a role in supporting babies who face particular challenges to become independent feeders earlier than might otherwise be possible. In this situation the device acts as a bridge, enabling the baby to feed himself while simultaneously developing the necessary skills. But the fact that a silicone feeder, for example, can perform a therapeutic function in one situation doesn't make it advisable for a baby who does not need it. Devices used unnecessarily tend to hinder developmental progress rather than support it.

Changing ideas about infant feeding

By the 1970s, babies in the US and the UK were generally being given their first pureed foods at or before 3 months of age; by the 1980s, this had moved to around 4 months. (Interestingly, because babies as young as this are rarely able to sit without significant support, it was considered acceptable to feed them in a semi-reclining position—which is now highlighted as being unsafe, since it increases the risk of choking.)

In the 1970s, it was usual to begin with rice cereal mixed with human milk or formula, moving on gradually to vegetables and then fruit. Meat, fish, and egg (yolks only, initially) were added from 6 months. Finger foods were introduced at around 9 months, alongside spoon feeding of increasingly thick purees and then mashes, in a staged approach. Scheduled reduction of breastfeeding was the norm, with the goal being complete weaning by 12 months. Parents were also advised to start with one meal a day and to offer their baby the same food for a three- to five-day trial period, in case of an adverse reaction.

Rice as a first food

For generations, the first food given to most babies in the US and the UK was rice cereal. Rice has long been a staple food in many parts of the world, so it is a plentiful and cheap ingredient—a point not lost even today on commercial baby food manufacturers. Rice was popular with doctors and parents because it provided calories and therefore stimulated weight gain (thought to be a good thing, even in excess). As a bland food, it was seen as being readily acceptable to (young) babies, easy to digest, and unlikely to trigger an allergic response. Over time, it was discovered to be lacking in many important micronutrients, notably iron, but, rather than being rejected as a suitable food for infants, it was simply "fortified." Ironically, this means that baby rice is often promoted as a good source of iron even though the iron in many other foods can be more readily absorbed. In recent years rice has been found to contain potentially high levels of heavy metals such as lead, arsenic, cadmium, and mercury;[10] it is also recognized as being highly processed. As a result, many health professionals are now actively opposed to its use as a regular weaning food.[11]

However, except for families where there is a strong history of allergy, such caution is not needed for babies of 6 months and older, whose digestive systems are more mature. Indeed, there is no evidence that it reduces the risk of allergies or food intolerances. What it does do is slow down the baby's exposure to new foods, thereby limiting the number he will be offered in his first year. This is important because it's common, when babies become toddlers, for them to start to dislike some foods, and to be fearful of foods they don't recognize (neophobia). A baby who enters toddlerhood with a narrow list of foods that he is happy to eat risks having a very limited diet if that list shrinks.

In 2002, the World Health Organization (WHO) recommended that babies should be exclusively breastfed from birth, with complementary foods introduced at "around six months," which is when their need for iron and zinc, in particular, can no longer be met reliably from their own body stores and their mother's milk.[12] The American Academy of Pediatrics followed suit a few years later, and this remains their recommendation today.[13] Since 2000, there has been an increasing emphasis on identifying signs of an individual baby's *developmental readiness* for solid foods—notably the ability to sit upright and an obvious interest in others' food. However, many doctors, nurses, and therapists still assume that purees and spoon feeding are the way to start, in spite of the fact that, at 6 months, they are not necessary as a first step. As the next chapter explains, baby-led weaning addresses this oversight.

LUKE'S STORY

Jill's account

LUKE'S HISTORY

Luke's mom is a pediatric dietitian and a fervent supporter of baby-led weaning. She followed BLW successfully with her first child and has since worked with families on implementing this approach. However, she found herself struggling when it came time to start solids with her second son, Luke.

Luke got off to a good start with breastfeeding but problems with weight gain and fussiness began to appear at around two months. He subsequently transitioned to bottle feedings of his mom's milk, together with reflux medications. When he started on solid foods, using a regular BLW approach, he gagged more than most babies and his mom became frightened to offer him food unless his dad was home. She connected with me through the Starting Solids Network (a network of professionals who are enthusiastic about BLW, to which we both belong), and I started to consult with her virtually.

LUKE'S FEEDING THERAPY INTERVENTION AND PROGRESS

I began working with Luke when he was around 8 months old. As I watched him eat I noticed that he appeared anxious, coughed when he got food pieces in his mouth, tried to engage with his mom to avoid eating, and, when given a pre-loaded spoon, would flip it to the nonfood end. We suspected that a posterior restrictive lingual frenulum, or tongue-tie, might be contributing to his struggles (this type is less easy to detect than an anterior one), but given the ongoing COVID-19 pandemic his mom was hesitant to have a tongue-tie assessment and possible release carried out.

Our initial sessions focused on therapeutic feeding techniques, such as using frozen straws and a silicone feeder to work on chewing and encouraging self-feeding with soft food strips like avocado. Our aim was to help Luke gain confidence and allow him time to develop better chewing skills before reintroducing foods that were harder to break down. Because he found lumpy textures particularly challenging we began offering him food teethers that he could gnaw on without having to deal with "bits," like a mango pit and a rib bone, as well as finely mashed soft foods from a pre-loaded spoon and from his tray. We also tried cup drinking, with slightly thinned purees, which Luke really enjoyed.

I encouraged Luke's parents to include him in family mealtimes, but they found that he sometimes became overwhelmed when everyone was at the table at the same time and wouldn't eat. So, I suggested that his mom start each meal by eating with him on her own for 15 to 20 minutes, to ensure he had some practice with foods that were challenging for him, and the chance to eat if he wanted to, before everyone else came to sit at the table.

From 9 to 12 months, we worked on Luke's chewing skills using large foods, like corn cobs with the kernels stripped off, as well as the silicone feeder and frozen straws. We also worked on getting him to take bites of meltable solids and soft solid strips, such as avocado. We offered him firm food strips dipped into purees and mashes and helped him transition to straw drinking using a therapeutic straw cup. Throughout, we concentrated on respecting his cues, eliminating all pressure to eat, eating with him, and using an "around the bowl" technique (see page 200) to help him get used to new foods. When we introduced smaller pieces of food we used only soft solids, such as sweet potato, as we noticed that he seemed unnerved by foods that didn't squish immediately in his mouth, preferring those that were meltable and easy to break down.

Luke continued to struggle with each new texture but would master it after a few weeks of practice. At 9 months he was seen in person by a second speech pathologist, who confirmed the presence of a posterior tongue-tie and gave Luke's mom a series of oral motor and therapeutic feeding activities to further encourage his chewing skills. By the time he turned a year old, his parents were feeling much more confident about his eating. His gagging had stopped and he was able to take bites from resistive food strips like cheese sticks, as well as soft solid strips and meltable solids. He was managing small pieces and could gnaw on a whole peeled peach. The last time I saw him, at 13 months, he was self-feeding a large variety of table foods and, while his mom felt he needed to continue refining his chewing skills, she was feeling confident about his progress and no longer required my coaching.

DISCUSSION

Tongue-tie is rightly seen as significant for breastfeeding but it can also cause difficulties during the transition to solid foods, owing to the need to move the tongue laterally to transfer food to the sides of the mouth for chewing. Luke's story illustrates the importance of diagnosing tongue-tie early. Had his condition been spotted when the breastfeeding difficulties first appeared, not only may he have been able to continue nursing, but his transition to solid foods may have been easier, too. I was impressed that his mom sought help, and with how she whole-heartedly implemented my suggestions even though she was already anxious about Luke's feeding himself. This must have been hard for her, given how committed she was to BLW, both professionally and as a parent. It was rewarding to be able to work with her, adapting BLW to turn Luke's solid feeding journey around, and I was delighted when she felt that they had gotten through the rough patch and no longer needed my support.

Luke's mom's perspective

As a pediatric registered dietitian, I thought that feeding my baby would be the easy part. My son started off his breastfeeding journey very smoothly. Then, at around 2 months, things started to get hard. He was feeding all the time! He was fussy, gassy, and his stools started to become green. We went on a dairy-free diet with some improvement but something was still not right. Weight gain became slow and we were struggling. He was feeding for short bursts every hour or two around the clock. I was working with a lactation consultant but, given the pandemic, it was all virtual. Luke would take a few sucks, pull off the breast and cry, and refuse to take any more. After some time we decided to switch to bottles and start a reflux medication. Both happened at the same time so it's hard to say what did the trick, but he took to the bottle, and volume intake and weight gain improved. I thought we were in the clear. Come 6 months, when we started solids via baby-led weaning, things did not go well. We experienced some pretty scary gags on multiple occasions with all textures and types of food. Given Luke's age we took a brief break to give him some time to mature more, but that did not help. Feeding became impossible and gave me a lot of anxiety. I knew what to feed my baby and how to feed my baby, but when traditional methods were not working, and safety was of concern, I knew I needed help. Discovering ABLW was our saving grace! What I love about the adapted baby-led weaning approach is that it aligns with core principles of how to feed a baby while meeting the baby where they are at. It uses alternative techniques yet still provides key feeding building blocks.

In working with Jill we discovered that Luke had a significant posterior tongue-tie that likely had been contributing to some of our feeding issues from the start. Although it didn't seem to be the only issue impacting his ability to manage solid foods, we worked to maximize his tongue function to promote the best feeding outcomes. We focused on self-feeding with mashes, baby spoons, starter food strips, and silicone feeders, and expanded on textures as Luke tolerated them. It was truly remarkable to see his progression and the gag and aversion decrease over time. With every step of the process Jill eased my anxiety and stress. I would often be nervous to try new shapes and textures, and she was so encouraging. When she suggested we have Luke hold foods I was hesitant at first, but it was remarkable to see how much he actually enjoyed it and was more receptive to food that way. Adapted baby-led weaning was life changing for us. We would not have overcome all of Luke's feeding aversions without it. Our son is now a great eater and loves food!

This is the origin of the term "complementary feeding." The American Academy of Pediatrics recommends that breast- or formula feeding should continue alongside complementary foods until at least the baby's first birthday,[1] while the World Health Organization favors breastfeeding for two years or longer.[2] The conventional approach to weaning puts the parent in charge of deciding the starting age, the speed of transition, and the date when milk feedings will end; baby-led weaning (BLW) allows the baby to make these decisions for herself. In this sense BLW is similar to Ellyn Satter's Division of Responsibility in Feeding, which revolves around the importance of the baby choosing what to eat, how much, and how quickly.[3] The main difference is that, in BLW, the baby feeds herself from the very beginning. Eating (or not) is literally in the baby's hands.

Baby-led weaning is rooted in typical infant development. It recognizes that, at the point when the baby is showing the conventional signs of readiness (sitting upright with minimal support and showing an interest in food), she is also able to grasp food, bring it to her mouth, and chew it. There is therefore no need for her to be spoon fed or to have her food pureed. Provided food is presented in sizes, shapes, and textures that allow her to pick it up and eat it, she will be able to feed herself, just as she was able to do at the breast when she was a newborn (see "Self-feeding as a continuum," page 33), honing her skills as she goes. The same underlying thinking can be applied to babies whose development is on a slower trajectory, so that their abilities (rather than their chronological age) form the basis for how they are supported to engage with solid food. This allows them to progress at their own pace rather than be compelled to follow a program that doesn't take account of their individual needs.

Self-feeding as a continuum

Babies whose development is typical self-feed from the get-go. They also regulate their own appetite, knowing when to eat, how much to eat, how quickly to eat, and when to stop eating. This is the essence of intuitive eating. Provided she is not affected by medication given during labor, a newborn baby will, when placed skin to skin on top of her mother, spontaneously crawl toward the breast and latch on to get milk. She doesn't need to "be fed" or to have her intake decided for her. If babies can do this at birth, and are able to eat independently later as toddlers, it is hard to imagine why, at the point when they start solid foods, they should suddenly need to have their feeding controlled by an adult. In fact, human babies, like the young of all other mammals, are more than capable of feeding themselves with solid foods, provided they are given the opportunity to do so at the time that is right for them. Babies with a history of low muscle tone, or complex medical or surgical problems, may not match their peers' progress at all stages but they are nevertheless born on this same self-feeding trajectory. They just need additional support and an extended time frame to achieve their potential.

The baby-led approach also recognizes that babies are able to regulate their intake of food according to their appetite, and that the amounts of additional food needed at the beginning of the weaning period are extremely small. This allows the emphasis to be on the baby's gaining experience with food, learning to match appearance with texture and flavor, and becoming familiar with an extensive list of foods (as many as 100 or more by age one).[4] This in turn minimizes the chances that any neophobia or pickiness arising in toddlerhood will seriously limit her diet or make mealtimes stressful. A diet consisting only of purees—especially store-bought varieties— cannot provide a comparable range of experience.

Baby-led weaning is often presumed to be just about babies' feeding themselves with chunks of food, but it encompasses much more than this activity. It includes shared mealtimes and healthy family food, and letting the baby control the speed with which family foods replace milk feedings. Most important, BLW centers on trust and respect: trust that the baby knows what, when, and how much she needs to eat; trust that she has the abilities and skills to match her needs and to keep herself safe; and respect for her choices and her natural desire to explore new things. It's an *approach* to the introduction of solid foods, not simply a method of feeding.

Many adults eat for a variety of reasons unconnected with hunger—to comfort themselves, for example, or because the clock says it's lunchtime—rather than because their body needs food. This tangling up of eating with emotions often has its roots in childhood experiences of being made to "clean your plate," "take one more bite for Grandma," or "eat your vegetables so you can have dessert." In BLW there is no bribery or coercion to persuade the baby to eat, and no praise or reward when she takes a bite. She eats because she is hungry, and because she's with her family, not in order to please her caregiver or to receive a treat.

No exaggeration, after the very first self-feed my twins did, I realized that I need to trust them more. Trust that they will eat what they can, trust they will try the foods, and trust that their bodies will protect them when they need it. It's hard to let go when all I want to do is make sure they are okay. But it's really rewarding to see that they are far more capable of handling difficult things than I thought.

Brie, mother of Liliana and Viviana,
born at 28 weeks' gestation

The practice of BLW fits right in with the science of child development, as well as with other research into infant feeding. For example, we know that children eat more when they are allowed to play with their food,[5] whereas pressure to eat tends to result in lower consumption.[6] We also know that children who are exposed to a variety of food textures from 6 months have better chewing skills at 12 months and 2 years than those who don't have this experience.[7] In particular, babies who are restricted to purees get less practice at moving their tongue from side to side[8]—possibly because purees don't trigger the tongue lateralization reflex in the same way that textured foods do. Consequently, when they eventually move on to pieces of food they often try to swallow each bite whole, rather than chew it. In spite of this accumulated knowledge, until 2012 there was almost no research into the BLW approach per se. Since then, the evidence has begun to build, such that we now know that BLW is associated with the following:

- more breastfeeding, for longer[9]
- the timely introduction of solid foods—at around 6 months[10]

- greater dietary variety, and a greater intake of fruit and vegetables, during the weaning period[11]
- a reduced desire for sweet foods[12]
- increased responsiveness to having eaten enough (satiety)[13]
- less fussiness and picky eating, and greater enjoyment of food[14]

We also know that BLW is no more likely than the conventional approach to result in adverse effects on energy intake or growth or to lead to an increased risk of choking or iron deficiency.[15] In addition, there are suggestions that it may help reduce the likelihood of obesity[16] and enhance the development of gross, fine motor, and language skills.[17] Some dental clinicians have found anecdotally that molar eruption begins earlier for babies who are chewing and gnawing on real foods from a young age, while many experts in orthodontics believe that early chewing enhances the growth of the bones and muscles of the face.[18] More research is needed but the signs are very positive.

How BLW works

In baby-led weaning, the baby is included in family mealtimes from as early as her parents wish—usually being held in their arms or on their lap. Once she can hold her head and trunk erect and reach out to grab things (typically at around 6 months) she is given the chance to begin exploring food. Seated in a high chair or on her parent's knee, she will have food placed in front of her on the tray or table or offered directly for her to take from her parent's hand. She is allowed all the time she needs to touch, squish, taste, smear, and generally get acquainted with the food, without being rushed or coerced into eating any particular item or amount.

Wherever possible the baby is offered a small selection of the same healthy, home-prepared food that the rest of the family is eating at that meal. The aim is to provide plenty of variety, with something from each food group over the course of a day, so that all the nutrients she is likely to need are available to her. The food is presented in strips, pieces, or wedges that she can grasp with her fist, with some sticking out for her to sniff, lick, and gnaw. In general, the texture needs to be soft enough for her to bite through with her gums but not so soft that she can't hold the piece easily. The exception is strips of meat, which, although too tough for most babies who are just starting out to bite and chew, are great for gnawing and for the flavorsome, iron-rich juice they contain. Very slippery foods are usually avoided at first, since they tend to be difficult to grasp and lead to frustration. Human milk or infant formula continues to be the baby's main source of nourishment for several months, with milk feedings offered as they have been, in and around the solid meals.

Most babies who are allowed to self-feed in this way eat very little or nothing on their first few encounters with food—and sometimes for several weeks. Since the baby's main source of nourishment will still be human milk or formula, there is no reason for this to cause concern, provided she is well and thriving. Indeed, in the beginning it's better that she is *not* hungry (or tired) before a meal, since she doesn't yet understand that solid food can fill her belly. A milk feed shortly before each solid meal is therefore a good idea. After several weeks of food discoveries and practice the baby will begin to eat more purposefully at mealtimes; the amounts will increase, and, as her dexterity improves, she will be able to manage smaller pieces. At this point small amounts of water can be offered in an open cup—enough to quench her thirst without reducing her appetite for milk feedings. Gradually, bowls, plates, and utensils will start to be included and milk feedings will begin to dwindle until, eventually, the baby—now a toddler—is relying on family food for all her nutrition.

> Adapted baby-led weaning helped me reframe the narrative that I, along with most parents, had in my mind of what meal time would be like with my baby. It went from stressing about how much food Skylar would consume, and for how long she would sit, to pressure-free meals that were more qualitative and *fun* (for both of us)!"
>
> Jaime, mother of Skylar, who had gastroesophageal reflux and FPIES

BLW and responsive feeding

The term *responsive feeding* is commonly used nowadays in relation to the feeding of babies and children. It can be thought of as one aspect of a wider philosophy of responsiveness within caregiving and parenting.[19] However, while baby-led weaning is an excellent fit with a responsive approach to caring for babies, it is not the same thing as responsive feeding. At its simplest, responsive feeding means responding to a child's cues that she is hungry and respecting her signals that she has eaten enough. In practice, this tends to mean

- feeding slowly and patiently, while maintaining eye contact[20]
- allowing the child to choose what to eat (from a selection prepared by the parent)[21]
- watching for signs that she is ready for the next bite, and not putting anything into her mouth without her permission[22]

There's no doubt that all of this makes eating much more pleasant than being cajoled, bribed, or forced to eat, or having food withheld—but it still allocates the active role to the caregiver rather than the child, reducing the opportunity for truly intuitive eating.

Baby-led weaning is different. It interprets "feeding" not as something done *to* the baby but as something done *by* her. The adult's role is to prepare the food appropriately to the child's skill level and make sure she can reach it easily. Once the baby starts eating, the only signals the caregiver needs to watch for are that she wants more food or that she has finished. Since the baby is in charge of each bite, her "permission" is not required and, provided she is not hurried, she naturally takes care of the "slowly, patiently" side of things by eating at her own chosen pace. Similarly, when her caregiver isn't pushing her to eat more than she wants, the meal ends when the baby chooses. When babies feed themselves, being responsive simply means being a good table companion.

Adapted baby-led weaning

Adapted BLW is a blend of BLW and responsive feeding. It takes self-feeding as the starting point, making the baby the active feeder, then adds targeted support, where and when it's needed. The overall goals are the same as in BLW but the way they are achieved is different. The practicalities of this approach are described in detail in chapters 7 and 8.

ABLW addresses the fact that babies who face feeding challenges commonly require a transitional phase before full self-feeding is possible. For example, they may find hand-to-mouth movements difficult. In this case the caregiver can provide responsive "facilitation" (see page 188) in a way that supports the baby as an active participant in the feeding process, rather than turning to spoon feeding as the only option. Similarly, there may be a need for bridge devices, such as silicone feeders, to help the baby develop handling and chewing skills. In this transitional phase, which may last for many weeks or months, pureed and mashed foods may also play a bigger role than they typically do in BLW. However, the underpinning principle remains the same: The process is led by the baby.

Apart from the targeted use of devices and facilitation, a key difference between adapted BLW and regular BLW is that the introduction of solid foods may need to begin later than 6 months (actual age, or adjusted to allow for prematurity), since the baby must be physically and developmentally ready to engage in the process, with strong foundational gross motor skills. However, as with regular BLW, the initial focus is on her exploring food using all her senses, rather than on eating. She will usually be engaged in touching, grasping, holding, sniffing, licking, and gnawing on food strips, gaining experience with both flavors and textures, for some weeks before she actually eats anything solid. During this time her milk feedings will continue to supply the majority of her nourishment (with vitamin and mineral supplements as necessary).

Adapted BLW is probably most effective when it forms part of individualized pre-feeding and therapeutic feeding programs (see pages 126 and 129), facilitated and overseen by a qualified feeding therapist. The selection and preparation of foods will be based on the baby's gross motor skills, dexterity, coordination, and oral motor skills, and the therapist will guide the caregivers as to appropriate shapes, size, and textures, to allow for safe eating and swallowing. As the baby's self-feeding skills develop, the amount of support she needs will lessen, until—like her typically developing peers—she is able to manage a large variety of foods safely and independently.

> What we know is that all babies benefit from responsive feeding practices, and a baby-led transition to solids is just that—a strategy that lets a baby take the lead, despite any additional challenges they may face.
>
> Kary Rappaport, and Kimberly Grenawitzke, pediatric occupational therapists

Benefits of adapted baby-led weaning

For babies whose feeding abilities are compromised, ABLW offers many benefits when compared with the conventional approach. First and foremost, the opportunity to feed herself engages the baby's interest and encourages her to play an active part rather than be passively compliant. In contrast to the usual dynamic at the start of complementary feeding, her attention is directed to the food, not to the caregiver. Sharing meals with the family gives her space to learn and provides role models whose behavior she can copy. It helps to build trusting relationships and make eating enjoyable for all. Looking down at food and reaching out to pick it up utilizes and strengthens the baby's core muscles and promotes eye-hand coordination.[23] Practice at taking food to her mouth helps with hand-to-mouth movements (as opposed to head-toward-food movements, which are common with spoon feeding), while holding large pieces of food with two hands, and passing them hand to hand, encourages what is known as midline orientation. This is important for learning to use both hands together, for visual focus, and for eye-hand coordination.

Early experience with a range of textures and foods that require chewing promotes side-to-side tongue movements, builds jaw strength, and teaches the baby to make rhythmic, appropriate-size (that is, "graded") up-down chewing and biting movements, known as munching. It facilitates desensitization for babies who may otherwise reject complex textures, helping them to recognize different foods and how they behave. It also helps them to sense where food is inside their mouth (oral proprioception) and begin to move it around purposefully. Chewing breaks down the food and mixes it with saliva, which contains digestive enzymes, creating a soft, mushy consistency. This makes it easier to pull together into a bolus and then swallow and starts the process of digestion.

Learning to chew effectively is especially important for babies who have anatomical disorders, sensory issues, or low muscle tone, since they are prone to swallowing unchewed or partially chewed pieces of food, which can lead to digestive difficulties and discomfort. In addition, although research into links between the development of chewing skills and the growth of the bones and muscles of the face and throat is scarce, it makes sense that they would be connected. Early chewing is therefore likely to be beneficial for a population of babies who are at risk for airway disorders. The bonus is that all of this functional activity can take place as part of a shared social event, at the family table. Experience suggests that babies whose development is atypical develop these important skills earlier with ABLW than with spoon feeding. They therefore gain independence with feeding at a younger age and, because they are exposed to a wide range of foods from the outset in an unpressured environment, they stand to reap long-term nutritional benefits.

> He was not just sitting there with his mouth open waiting for the next spoonful; he was active, engaged, and involved with this very important aspect of life. He was using his hands, lips, tongue, teeth, and willpower during each mealtime. He and his therapist have taught me so much.
>
> Jill, grandmother of Ethan, who has Down syndrome

HENRY'S STORY

Jill's account

HENRY'S HISTORY

Henry's mom is a pediatric nurse in a children's hospital. Henry is her second child. He was born with a restrictive lingual frenulum, or tongue-tie, which was released at three days by an ear, nose, and throat specialist (ENT). A few days later a dentist carried out the release of an upper-lip tie. Henry was breastfed until he was 3 weeks old, when repeated episodes of choking at the breast forced his mom to switch to giving him her milk by bottle. At 5 weeks, he underwent a fiberoptic endoscopic evaluation of swallowing (FEES) and was diagnosed with moderate to severe laryngomalacia (low laryngeal muscle tone), with accompanying problems controlling milk inside his mouth, difficulty swallowing (dysphagia), and reflux. When he was 2 months, corrective surgery (supraglottoplasty) was recommended. However, having discussed the pros and cons with their pediatrician, his parents opted to defer the surgery until Henry was older.

From around this time, and on the recommendation of the children's hospital, Henry's parents began to give him combined feeds of his mom's milk and formula (half and half), in order to achieve a slightly thicker consistency. They found that feeding him lying on his side, and pacing the feeding, helped him manage the flow of the milk. He was prescribed courses of medication to control the reflux, but, in the periods when he was not taking it, feedings could last up to 45 minutes because he would constantly stop and start. His parents often had to break his feeding into shorter sessions in order to get him to finish a six-ounce bottle.

Henry was rapidly developing a feeding aversion, and feedings were becoming very stressful.

Henry continued to receive his mom's milk until he was 4 months old. He had repeat FEES at 2.5 months and 4 months. The first and second FEES showed liquid going deep into his larynx, indicating a weakness in the swallowing mechanism. While aspiration of fluid into his lungs was not observed, it could not be ruled out.

HENRY'S FEEDING THERAPY INTERVENTION AND PROGRESS

I met Henry when he was 7.5 months old. In view of the difficulty he was having with bottle feedings, his mom wanted to know how to approach the transition from purees to solid foods as safely as possible. She had already worked with two other feeding therapists but had not found their input helpful. At this point Henry was having two meals a day, at breakfast and lunch, both fed to him by spoon. (His parents had stopped offering him dinner, as he would then refuse his bottle, and they were concerned about his calorie intake.) He would have oatmeal mixed with formula at breakfast and a vegetable or fruit puree at lunch. On one occasion, his parents gave him a whole banana to gnaw on but he caught a virus shortly afterward and subsequently refused to eat banana, so they abandoned the idea.

At our first session, Henry would not pick up food or bring it to his mouth. He did accept a small amount of a vegetable puree when it was fed to him from a spoon and then accepted the same puree, thinned with formula, from an open cup, with assistance. He also drank a little of the same thinned puree through a therapeutic straw cup when it was held for him. At the conclusion of the session, I recommended using responsive feeding techniques to address Henry's feeding aversion, and capitalizing on what he liked (for example, thinned purees from the cup) to help him see eating as a positive experience. I also recommended using pre-loaded spoons and a silicone feeder to offer him purees and soft solid food mashes, to introduce more texture. I suggested frozen straws and food popsicles, as well as starter food strips, to get him to bring food to his mouth, allow him to explore food without pressure, and stimulate chewing practice. I explained the benefits of family mealtimes for modeling eating behavior and of having all the food on the table, family-style, prior to everyone sitting down, so that the meal was not interrupted.

When I saw Henry two weeks later, his parents were implementing my suggestions at three mealtimes each day. Progress was slow, since he definitely preferred for someone else to feed him. He was hit or miss with self-feeding of food strips: His mom would sometimes have to hold the strip first and then he would take it from her hand rather than picking it up from the high chair tray. Despite this, he gradually started to accept more textured purees from the spoon, although he would frequently spit food out.

Over the next two weeks Henry's parents continued to persevere with starter strips like carrot, pepper, celery, and meat strips, and with pre-loaded spoons and the silicone feeder. He was now willing to bring food such as grilled chicken strips to his mouth but he occasionally bit off a large chunk. His mom was concerned about choking and that this might exacerbate his aversion, so she used the silicone feeder for these harder-to-break-down foods. There was a minor setback when Henry was discovered to have an egg allergy, but there was no mistaking the fact that his willingness to feed himself was growing.

At the time of writing Henry is 9 months old; therapy is ongoing, and progress continues to be steady.

DISCUSSION

In seven weeks, Henry went from two meals a day, where he was accepting only spoon fed purees, to self-feeding table-food mashes from a pre-loaded spoon three times a day, and gnawing on steak, lamb chops, and a variety of starter strips. His ABLW therapy journey has only just begun, but the change from adult-directed to baby-led feeding occurred quickly. With continued work on refining his chewing skills, and coaching for his family on how to progress safely with different food sizes, shapes, and textures, the future is bright.

Henry's mom's perspective

Our sweet little boy Henry was born just over two weeks early, at a gestation of 37 weeks and 5 days. Our journey began at birth when the lactation consultant in the hospital diagnosed Henry with a lip- and tongue-tie on day one. He had both releases done by 10 days old and breastfeeding was going well. Around 3 weeks old, Henry developed stridor (a high-pitched sound while breathing), both at rest and when breastfeeding. He had trouble transferring milk and his weight gain was reduced. Our pediatrician recommended we see a speech pathologist and ENT to have him evaluated for suspected laryngomalacia. Craniosacral therapy was also recommended by our pediatric dentist after the tongue and upper lip release, to help with feeding while we waited to see the ENT, and we began this when Henry was approximately 4 weeks old. Henry had his first FEES at 5 weeks old, which confirmed the pediatrician's suspicion. The doctors recommended that I start pumping and thickening my milk with formula, along with pace-feeding Henry in a side-lying position. We also started reflux medication twice a day at this point. Over the next three months Henry had two additional FEES, which showed that milk was going deep into his larynx during feeding, and we were followed closely by both the ENT and the speech pathologist. We went to several different speech pathologists for feeding therapy, with no success. Bottle feeding continued to be a roller coaster, with some good days followed by more bad days. Some days we were literally force-feeding him, just to get the minimum daily requirement of ounces in. We tried five different formulas before finding one that worked. My husband and I were desperate for some relief for ourselves and our son. We were constantly questioning if we had made the right decision in refusing the surgical route.

Fast forward to 6 months old, and we decided to start purees. Little did we know that Henry had developed aversions from all the feeding troubles over the past six months. It was a slow start and he didn't seem to enjoy any type of food. He did tons of gagging, coughing, or just flat-out refusing of food—we felt so defeated and had no idea what to do. When Henry was around 7 months old my colleague recommended we consult with Jill. We were desperate and decided to try feeding therapy one more time. When I met with Jill I felt immediate relief. She presented a type of feeding, called adapted baby-led weaning, that has now changed our lives. I was hesitant at first because of Henry's trouble swallowing, but my husband and I made the decision to move forward cautiously. At first, Henry continued to refuse to bring anything to his mouth but would accept an open cup with a nectar-thick puree-water mix (IDDSI level 2) and straws with frozen puree inside, if a caregiver held it for him. We celebrated the little wins and continued trying. We followed his lead and worked on strengthening his jaw with raw foods like strips of carrot, cucumber, and sweet peppers. After a few weeks he began bringing large pieces of food, like strips of steak, lamb chop bones, cooked sweet potatoes, raw vegetables, and some table mashes, to his mouth. The first time he brought the steak to his mouth, I literally cried tears of joy—my baby was eating and truly enjoying it. There was finally a light at the end of the tunnel. We did hit another bump in the road when Henry had an allergic reaction to eggs at almost 9 months old. I had always considered that it was possible he had a food allergy that was contributing to all of his feeding struggles; it was just never confirmed. It's another piece of the puzzle.

Henry is now a little over 9 months old and we are still working on solids and table mashes, but this method of feeding has made mealtime fun again in our home and has changed our expectations for our son's future into one that includes a healthy relationship with food.

3
·····

How Babies
Learn to Eat

In order to appreciate the difficulties faced by babies whose responses and abilities in relation to eating develop differently, we need first to understand how feeding skills develop in typical situations. This chapter describes the interplay of reflexes, motor skills, and the sensory system that enables babies born at term, with no underlying physical or neurological obstacles, to feed themselves—first via breast or bottle and then as part of shared family mealtimes.

The origins of feeding skills

The majority of babies are born able to feed themselves with milk. Like the young of other mammals, they are guided by instinct to find their mother's nipple, latch on, and feed. But the innate abilities that enable them to do this are not skills the baby has learned—they are reflex actions, triggered primarily by smell and touch. Some of these reflexes produce feeding behaviors while others serve a protective function. Together, they help babies survive and thrive. Reflex movements happen automatically, without any intention—and they can't be voluntarily overridden. Think of your own knee-jerk reflex as an example. Reflexes are often tested for, at any age, as evidence that the brain and nervous system are properly functioning. Over the first few months after a baby is born, some of his reflexes (like the rooting reflex) disappear completely, while others (like coughing) continue unchanged throughout life. A few (swallowing, for example) continue as both reflexive and voluntary movements. But the majority of those related to feeding, such as the sucking reflex, become integrated into the baby's growing portfolio of acquired skills, meaning that the movement itself persists but under voluntary control, rather than as an involuntary reflex.

Commonly, seven reflexes are described in relation to feeding in young babies: the rooting reflex, the suckling/sucking reflex, the swallowing reflex, the tongue-thrust (or "extrusion") reflex, the transverse tongue reflex, the gag reflex, and the phasic bite reflex. All of these relate to the mouth and/or throat. However, there are now known to be a further twenty reflexes, involving other parts of the body, that are also connected with early feeding behavior.[1] Some reflexes in both these groups continue to be important to feeding effectiveness and safety well beyond the newborn period—as does the cough reflex, which is frequently overlooked in relation to feeding. Altogether, there are ten reflexes that are relevant to how babies navigate the introduction of solid foods.

- **The palmar grasp reflex:** The baby closes his fist in response to an object touching his palm.
- **The hand-to-mouth reflex:** The baby brings his hand to his mouth in response to having his cheek or palm stroked.
- **The rooting/mouth gape reflex:** The baby turns or tilts his head toward a stimulus (such as the breast or bottle) when his face is touched, simultaneously opening his mouth wide.
- **The suckling/sucking reflex:** The baby sucks in response to pressure of the breast or nipple (or a finger) against his palate.
- **The swallowing reflex:** A sequence of contractions of the muscles of the larynx and pharynx, triggered when food, liquid, or saliva reaches the back of the throat, to move it into the esophagus. It can also be triggered by suckling.
- **The transverse tongue reflex (also known as the lateral tongue reflex):** A sideward movement of the tongue toward the stimulus, in response to touch (finger, toy, food) or taste.
- **The phasic bite reflex:** Opening and closing of the jaw in response to a finger or food being placed on the chewing surface of the gums.
- **The tongue-thrust/extrusion reflex:** When his lip or the tip of his tongue is touched, the baby pushes his tongue outward and forward.
- **The gag reflex:** Elevation of the back part of the tongue and contraction of the pharyngeal muscles and the esophagus in a retching/pre-vomiting movement. The effect is to shut off the airway and esophagus and propel

the object forward to prevent both swallowing and inhalation.

- **The cough reflex:** Forced expulsion of air from the lungs, in response to food or an object detected at the entrance to the oropharynx (or beyond), aimed at clearing the airway.

Many of the skills that relate to self-feeding have their origins in these very early reflexes. They can be considered under six headings: oral skills (involving the mouth and throat), sensory development, manual dexterity (fine motor), posture and movement (gross motor), protective mechanisms, and advanced eating skills.

The development of oral feeding skills

The development of basic, foundational oral feeding skills begins in the womb. At 4 weeks after conception, when the baby is still an embryo, he already has an identifiable tongue, and by as early as 6 weeks he is beginning to swallow. Suckling movements are evident from around 12 weeks, with sucking to support feeding possible from around 32 weeks and effective coordination of suck-swallow-breathe usual by 36 weeks.

Toward the end of a full-term pregnancy, conditions in the womb get a little cramped. This means that the baby is forced to curl up. As a result, when he is born he naturally assumes a curled-up position, known as physiological flexion. This natural flexion of his body and neck provides stability for his movements, making him better able to latch and suckle.[2] It also makes it easier for him to bring his hand to his mouth, which in turn triggers rooting, mouth opening, and suckling.

When a newborn baby's nose, lips, or cheek touch the skin of his mother's breast, he will "root" toward the nipple, turning his head and opening his mouth. As he does this his tongue will reach down and forward to help draw in the breast, shaping itself with a central groove running from front to back, to help transport the milk to his throat for swallowing. The presence of fatty "sucking" pads in his cheeks helps to reduce space inside his mouth and stabilize the nipple. The touch of the breast on the baby's tongue and/or palate stimulates the suckling reflex, in which his tongue compresses and massages the breast with a peristaltic, forward–backward wavelike motion known as suckling. (Babies feeding from a bottle or sucking on a pacifier use a similar technique, but with more emphasis on creating a vacuum to draw the milk in, and a less well-defined rhythm.[3]) When he is effectively latched, the newborn will feed in a coordinated suckle-swallow-breathe pattern, with a swallow after each suckle.

Breastfeeding skills: sequence of events

In the newborn period, feeding at the breast involves a unique series of actions:

- The baby searches for the breast with head-turning and bobbing movements.
- The baby's mouth opens wide and his head tilts back.
- The baby's tongue lowers and comes forward to the lower gum/lip (or beyond), developing a groove running centrally from front to back.
- The baby's chin, tongue, and lower lip make contact with the breast.

- The breast (including the nipple) is drawn in and stabilized between the tongue, fatty pads in the cheeks, and the palate.

- The baby's lips form a seal around the breast with the upper lip passively positioned and the lower lip turned out.

- The tongue maintains steady contact with the breast and moves rhythmically forward and backward; at the same time, the baby lowers and raises his lower jaw, with deep jaw excursions, to create a vacuum and facilitate compression of the breast between the tongue and palate (suckling).

- As the breast is compressed, milk flows into the baby's mouth and triggers a swallow.

- The baby feeds in a relaxed way, breathing through his nose; the breast tissue may be seen to move slightly but the shape of the breast does not alter.

Over the first 4 to 6 months, suckling evolves into sucking, which is a more mature action, with greater upward movement of the tongue and more active use of the lips.[4] At the same time, the reflexive element fades, along with the rooting reflex. This helps explain why the parents of a breastfeeding baby of 3 months who is nursing well may not be able to persuade him to drink from a bottle, since the integration of these reflexes means he can no longer be "tricked" into sucking by having the bottle nipple rubbed against the roof of his mouth. Breastfeeding babies continue to use the familiar suckling action at the breast because it is more effective than sucking at removing the milk, but it becomes integrated into a voluntary sequence of movements. At around 2 to 3 months, as the baby gains greater control over the movements of his mouth, he becomes able to sustain longer bouts of breast- or bottle feeding without needing to pause.

The swallowing reflex is present from as early as 15 weeks' gestation.[5] It is triggered when amniotic fluid, saliva, or milk reaches the back of the throat, as well as by suckling. As the larynx rises, the epiglottis tilts downward, covering the entrance to the trachea and diverting milk away from the airway. Sucking, swallowing, and breathing need to be coordinated to allow the baby to remain oxygenated and to prevent him inhaling milk into his lungs (known as aspiration). This coordination happens spontaneously in a baby whose development is typical. In addition, young babies are protected from aspiration by the closeness of the epiglottis to the tip of the soft palate (see the following diagram—in a newborn, these will likely be touching). This prevents milk from spilling over into the trachea before the baby is ready to swallow.

As babies grow, and as they exercise their oral and facial muscles, their anatomy gradually changes. By about 4 months there is a noticeable difference in the relationship between the various structures of the mouth and throat, with the neck having lengthened and the larynx descended. This means that the epiglottis no longer provides the same degree of protection to the airway. In addition, by 4 to 6 months the stabilizing fatty sucking pads have disappeared from the baby's cheeks. Most babies are able to feed effectively without these extra safety features because they now have greater control of their tongue and jaw movements. However, these physical changes may

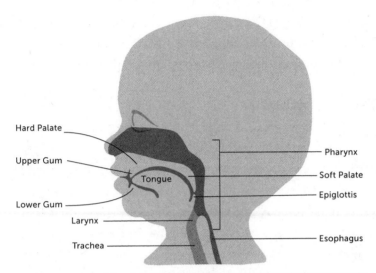

ANATOMICAL STRUCTURES RELATED TO SWALLOWING IN YOUNG BABIES

temporarily make aspiration more of a risk for babies whose development is atypical.

Two reflexes that are present from birth but come into their own as solid foods are introduced are the transverse (or lateral) tongue reflex and the phasic bite reflex. The transverse tongue reflex is activated when there is stimulation of one side of the tongue. This causes the tongue to move toward the stimulus, which will later be important for moving pieces of food from the center to the side of the mouth for chewing. The transverse tongue reflex is present until at least 9 months and may persist as late as 24 months. Mature tongue lateralization, in which the movement is intentional and controlled, begins to emerge at around 7 or 8 months.

The phasic bite reflex is the spontaneous opening and closing of the jaw in response to a finger or food placed on the chewing surface of the gums—like a gentle biting movement. This reflex diminishes between 9 and 12 months, when the baby has developed more controlled biting patterns.

Learning to chew

Chewing is a more complex skill than many people imagine; in fact, it's several skills in one. It involves the jaws, tongue, and cheek muscles acting together, in a series of repeated, refined, differentiated, and coordinated movements that process the food to make it ready for swallowing. Strictly speaking, babies don't *learn* to chew—they naturally begin to make chewing movements as their phasic bite reflex becomes integrated. However, they do need to *practice* chewing in order to expand and refine their skills, and to be able to manage a variety of textures easily.

The parts of the upper and lower jaw that protrude inside our mouth provide us with biting and chewing surfaces—first gums and, later, teeth. The anterior (front) portions of both jaws are used for taking off a piece of food or accepting a bite from an eating utensil such as a spoon, fork, or pair of chopsticks; the lateral (side) parts, which extend backward inside our cheeks, are for chewing. As adults, we have differently shaped teeth in these two distinct areas: the incisors at the front, for biting and cutting, and the premolars and molars in the back, for chewing. When babies are ready to start solid foods, some may already have one or two incisors, but they don't yet have molars, so their "lateral chewing surfaces" are their gums. However, it's useful for those caring for babies who need extra support with eating to be able to visualize where the baby's molars will erupt, in order to help him learn to chew effectively.

When adults take a bite of food with their incisors, they move it to their molars for chewing using backward and sideways movements of the tongue, with their buccal (cheek) muscles acting as a brake to keep the food in the right spot. Next they apply a combination of up-down munching movements, followed by circular grinding movements, to break the food down into progressively smaller pieces. As the smaller pieces accumulate, they use their tongue to catch them and direct them back to the molars for another go. They also do occasional sweeps to search for stray pieces in the cheeks and inside the lips and bring them back to join the rest, so that the whole mouthful is processed at more or less the same rate. When they sense that enough chewing has taken place, they use their tongue to collect the food together into a bolus and propel it backward for swallowing. This complex set of skills takes time and practice to develop. In babies, simple up-and-down munching is usually seen from around 12 weeks. Over the next few months these movements mature through lateral, diagonal, and finally circular (rotary) chewing actions. Rotary chewing can be seen as early as 18 months and is usually an acquired skill by around 24 months.[6] However, anecdotal evidence suggests it may appear much earlier in babies who feed themselves with pieces of food from the beginning of complementary feeding rather than being given purees. This may be simply because they have more practice at chewing than babies who are predominantly spoon fed, or because purees tend to spread around the inside of the mouth and don't trigger the transverse tongue reflex. Alternatively, it may be linked to the fact that handling food is thought to help us to predict how it will feel and behave inside our mouth.[7]

Did you know?

Chewing starts the digestive process not just by breaking the food into smaller particles to make it easier to swallow but by mixing those particles with saliva. Saliva contains the enzyme amylase, which begins the breakdown of starchy carbohydrates. Chewing—especially of crunchy foods— is also linked to pleasure centers in the brain, making it something we want to keep doing. So, chewing is good for digestion and enjoyment of food, as well as for safety.

Closely related to chewing are the skills associated with jaw grading, which rely on jaw stability and more refined muscular control. Graded jaw movements consist of fine, even, repetitive opening and closing movements—such as the gnawing-type action a baby might use to shave slivers off a whole, peeled apple—while graded jaw strength refers to the ability to apply the appropriate amount of pressure to bite through foods of different textures or firmness—a banana versus a cracker, for example. A third skill, that of grading bite size, involves gauging how wide to open the mouth in order to take bites from foods of contrasting thickness; for example, a chunk of peach and a thin strip of banana. These skills can help lay the foundation for later speech development as well as being important for managing foods of different sizes and more complex shapes and textures.

As adults, we tend to take graded biting and chewing for granted, but we only know that more force is required to bite through a stick of celery than a piece of avocado because we have learned it through experience; babies of 6 months are ready to start making these discoveries. There is some evidence that self-feeding may contribute to effective jaw grading.[8] Certainly, like rotary chewing, jaw grading is reported anecdotally as becoming refined earlier in babies who have been allowed to feed themselves with foods of different shapes and sizes from the beginning, when compared with those who have become conditioned to same-size spoonfuls fed to them by someone else.

At birth, the anatomical structures connected with feeding work as one: When the newborn baby roots for the breast, he moves his head, jaw, and tongue simultaneously. As he gets older and gains control over his movements he discovers, for example, how to bite on a food strip at the side of his mouth without at the same time turning his head toward it, and how to close his lips to make swallowing easier and prevent food from escaping while he chews. With practice, and exposure to a variety of food textures and shapes, he figures out how to move a small piece of food from the center to the side of his mouth for chewing; by 12 to 14 months, he will have developed sufficient control over the tip of his tongue to enable him to collect crumbs scattered around the inside of his mouth and dislodge food caught in his teeth or cheeks. This process of developing, refining, and differentiating movement of the tongue, lips, and jaw for biting and chewing is known as dissociation.

The skill of drinking from an open cup emerges in a similar way: To begin with, the baby uses his jaw and tongue together, typically biting on the cup, opening his mouth too wide, and using his tongue to suck the liquid in. With practice, he will be able to stabilize his jaw without moving it and hold his tongue in position inside his mouth to collect the liquid and take it back for swallowing. As jaw stability increases, babies become able to use their lips in isolation for more refined movements, such as pursing them around a straw, or closing them over a finger to suck off a dollop of yogurt. This level of dissociation is a prerequisite for speech development and the articulation of increasingly complex sounds.[9]

Sensory development

The senses play a key role in eating, from birth onward. A newborn baby uses vision, hearing, smell, taste, and touch to help him locate and recognize his mother's breast, and to latch on and feed. From then on his senses help him build a database of information that he will draw on throughout his life, not least when he begins the move to solid food. When we think about the senses in relation to eating, the one that springs to mind first tends to be taste. This is no surprise, given what a crucial role it plays in our liking—and disliking—of different foods. Taste develops very early (along with smell, which is closely related): Both the amniotic fluid that surrounds the baby in the womb and his mother's milk vary in flavor according to what she eats, so babies start to experience different flavors as soon as they can swallow. It's thought that these early flavor exposures influence their taste preferences months later, when they begin eating solid foods.[10]

All the senses have a part to play in the run-up to the introduction of solid foods, but the one that is most easily overlooked is touch—how we interpret what things feel like. We
have touch receptors in the lining of the oral cavity and in our
skin, which relay information to the brain about the tactile (or
haptic) features of the things we touch or that touch us. Our
hands, lips, and tongue are especially sensitive, suggesting
that we are meant to pay attention to touch when we're eating.
Indeed, research has shown that children are more likely to
reject food on the basis of its "feel" than either its flavor or its
appearance.[11] The haptic features of food include size, shape,
and texture. Size and shape are fairly straightforward qualities,
but texture is more complex: It covers not only basic attributes
such as hard/soft, wet/dry, and hot/cold but also the features
that dictate how the food will behave when it's grasped or
chewed. Is it juicy, rubbery, or crumbly? Does it dissolve, break
up, or become sticky? Does it have one texture on the outside
and another on the inside?

Our sense of touch is closely related to our sense of movement, or "proprioception," which tells us how our body is positioned and how the various parts relate to one another. As we
gain control over our muscles, touch and proprioception work
together to enable us to make purposeful movements even
when we can't see what we're doing. A baby relies strongly on
these two senses to feed himself effectively and safely. They
help him figure out how to close his hand around a piece
of food, how firmly to grasp it, how to guide it between his
lips, how to bite through it, how to move it around inside his
mouth, how to chew it effectively, and how to gather it up and

propel it backward in order to swallow it. Think about how you learned to hold a raspberry without crushing it, or bite into a cracker, and you will see that the only way for babies to fine-tune their skills is for them to explore food for themselves. It therefore makes sense to expose babies and young children to a wide variety of sizes, shapes, and textures—as well as flavors—during the weaning period.

Mouth mapping

When a baby breastfeeds, the breast fills his mouth and molds itself to the shape of the oral cavity. This means that all the baby can feel inside his mouth is the breast. During rest periods and sleep, his mouth will usually be closed, with his tongue resting in the hard palate; see Cassius, photo 4. (An open-mouth resting posture may be indicative of low orofacial muscle tone, a structural variance such as a high-arched palate or tongue-tie, an allergy or nasal congestion, or narrow nasal passages.[12] It may also be associated with sleep apnea.) However, when he is awake his tongue will be free to touch his lips, gums, and cheeks, as well as whatever other objects make their way to his mouth.

The feedback the baby gets from moving his tongue, fingers, teethers, and toys around inside his mouth promotes "oral somatosensory awareness,"[13] or a sense of what the inside of his mouth feels like. This in turn enables him to build a mental image of its internal dimensions and shape—that is, to "map" the inside of his mouth. At the same time, experience with a variety of toys and teethers, especially those with large protruding parts of different shapes, sizes, and textures, which provide deep pressure input, helps him match finger-feel with mouth-feel, and begins to desensitize his gag reflex.[14] Babies Grace, Simone, and Owen (photos 1, 2, and 3) are engaged in this sort of exploratory behavior. As he transitions to solid foods, this experience will help the baby judge how big a bite of food to take, how much pressure to exert in order to break it down, and how to maneuver it inside his mouth in order to chew it effectively and prepare it for swallowing. It will also enable him to detect when something is not right or needs a different approach, for example, when his gums are sore or when a bite of food consists of more than one texture. As he gets older this skill will become refined, enabling him, for example, to locate an unexpected fish bone and remove it safely.

Generalized mouthing of hands and fingers may be evident from 2 months, when the baby is lying on his tummy (prone), and from 3 months when on his back (supine). This matures into more discriminative mouthing, focusing on fingers and objects, by around 5 months.[15] By 6 months, the baby is ready to expand his experience into the world of food and to add temperature and taste to the mix of new sensations.

The development of manual dexterity

For a baby to make use of his developing oral feeding skills he first has to be able to get food to his mouth. Although this is largely done for him in the early days of breast- and bottle feeding, there are several reflexes that support his position at the breast, enabling him to latch on and feed in a relaxed way. Of these, two in particular will assist the transition to solid foods as they become integrated. They are the palmar grasp and hand-to-mouth reflexes.

Newborn babies spontaneously close their fist around objects that touch their palm. This means that when their hand touches their mother's breast, they gain an awareness of its shape and texture. This helps to orient the baby and provides some stability, while at the same time stimulating the production and flow of milk. The baby may actually knead his mother's breast while he is feeding, to trigger the milk ejection (or "let-down") reflex. Newborn babies also spontaneously take their hand to their mouth when either their cheek or hand is stimulated. This, too, helps to orient them at the breast, as well as cuing their caregiver that they may be hungry. Both reflexes disappear soon after 3 months and are replaced by more purposeful reaching, grasping, and mouthing. Grasping and hand-to-mouth movements gradually become integrated in parallel with the increasing sharpness of the baby's vision, as well as his ability to tilt his head up and down. This facilitates coordination of eyes, hands, and mouth, which in babies whose development follows a typical path is usually well defined by about 4 months.

As well as contributing to effective jaw grading, the action of bringing food to the mouth has been shown to play a role in helping coordinate the buildup to swallowing.[16] However, because the 6-month-old baby is used to taking his *hand* to his mouth, he is inclined to hit himself on the forehead with whatever is sticking out of his hand. Practice leads to a gradual adjustment of his aim, so that the object itself makes contact with his mouth. This fine-tuning is perfect for locating, picking up, and eating solid foods and is, in turn, prompted by those actions. It is usually well advanced by 6 months but will continue to mature after that.

At 6 months, the baby still uses his palm and fingers together to grasp things and is unable to open his fist voluntarily. This is why the first finger foods need to be graspable in his whole hand, with some sticking out (see photos 16, 17, 20, 21, 32, 33, 36, 69, and 70). By 7 to 8 months, the baby is starting to release things from his fist on purpose, meaning that he may be able to manage smaller chunks of food. Gradually, he begins to use his fingers and thumb independently, rather than his whole hand. With practice, this becomes refined so that, by 8 to 9 months he is able to isolate his forefinger and use it to point, poke, and scrape. This is quickly followed by the ability to pick up small objects and pieces of food, such as individual peas—and, later, individual grains of rice—between the tips of his forefinger and thumb, in what is known as the pincer grasp (as demonstrated by Adira and Owen in photos 46 and 47 and by Faith in photo 72).

The development of gross motor skills

The development of the large (gross) muscles of the body in the first 6 months is key to safe and effective self-feeding, both during that period and afterward. If a baby is to reach out and grasp pieces of food, chew and swallow safely, and use a spoon or cup, he must be able to maintain a stable sitting position while turning his head and moving his arms. In addition, he needs to be able to bring his hands together in midline at the front of his body, so that he can use both hands for a single task, such as turning over a piece of food or holding a cup. All of this requires strong core muscles and the ability to adapt his posture in order to stay balanced. Control over the smaller (distal) muscles of the body is always preceded by control of the larger and more central (proximal) muscles, so a strong core is a prerequisite for coordination and fine movements of the hands and fingers. Spending waking time, from birth onward, in a variety of positions—including upright (for example, against an adult's chest), on his tummy (prone), on his side, as well as on his back (supine)—facilitates development of the necessary strength and range of movement in the muscles of the neck, back, shoulders, arms, and legs. At the same time, interacting with people and being offered a variety of interesting objects to look at and handle stimulates the baby to attempt increasingly complex movements, so extending his skill range.

It's crucial not to underestimate the importance of gross motor development and its impact on establishing the foundational base for feeding skills. The transition from a newborn with little control of his body to a 6-month-old who can sit up and bring food to his mouth is a dynamic change. Many of the motor skills acquired during this time are related to self-feeding in more than one way. For example, pushing up on the hands when prone not only strengthens a range of core muscles—including the shoulders, which are important for reaching—it also provides sensory and pressure input to the hands. This encourages strength in the palm and fingers, leading to improved dexterity and grasping ability, while also stimulating the baby to pay attention to his hand movements. This will later help him to switch, for example, between the actions and effort needed to hold a slice of watermelon, and the more refined, pincer movement required to pick up a small crumb.

The impact of "container culture"

One aspect of modern life that can impact the development of the foundational motor skills that are so important for the timely and safe introduction of solid foods is the widespread use of "containers," such as baby seats, swings, rockers, and bassinets. With babies spending less time on the ground or in a parent's arms, and more time in rigid and constricting containers, we are seeing changes in head shape and a shift in the ages at which babies are meeting key developmental milestones. This is sometimes referred to as "container baby syndrome."

In the first few months of life, some babies spend almost no time either on their tummy or being carried upright. This can lead to a flattened back of the skull, with the potential to impact the growth of the face and jaw.[17] Being supine or in a seat that restricts movement can also inhibit the development of the muscles of the arms, shoulders, neck, and back, which are naturally exercised when babies lie on their tummy and lift their head and trunk off the ground. Some babies spend long periods in bouncers, standers, and walkers that force them to adopt positions for which they are not developmentally ready, with the potential to disrupt, and possibly delay, the normal development of muscles and joints.

It's not just about cribs and seats: Swaddling is also a form of containment. While being swaddled can be comforting when babies are distressed, having their arms restricted means they aren't able to bring their hands to their mouth. This reduces the opportunities for mouthing and mouth mapping (see "Mouth mapping," page 64), both of which are important for the development of feeding skills. In addition, swaddling during breastfeeding can make latching more difficult because it prevents the baby from using his hands to locate the breast and position himself. Even mittens, which are often used to prevent infants from scratching their face, interfere with normal feeding and mouthing behavior, as well as limiting the feedback babies should be getting from touching their body and the surfaces around them.

Hand-to-mouth activity is essential for feeding and crucial to a baby's wider development.[18] The hands and mouth have more sensory nerve endings than any other part of the body, and a baby's instinct is to use them together to learn about his world. Without feedback from hands and mouth combined, all aspects of a baby's development are at risk of being compromised. We need to think carefully about the potential long-term effects of restricting babies' movements.

Protective mechanisms related to eating

In addition to the seven reflexes that trigger feeding behaviors, there are two—the tongue-thrust reflex and the cough reflex—that exist primarily to protect the baby rather than to assist with eating. A third, the gag reflex, likely offers both protection and assistance.

The tongue-thrust reflex

The tongue-thrust reflex is present from birth. It occurs when something touches the tip of the baby's tongue or lips. The tongue responds by pushing outward and forward, ejecting the offending finger, blanket, spoon, or piece of food. This is thought to be a protection against anything other than a breast (or bottle nipple) getting into the mouth of a baby who is too immature to be able to deal with it. It is a mechanism that works both to protect the airway and to prevent the ingestion of anything inappropriate. The reflex typically fades between 4 and 6 months and is gradually replaced by more purposeful thrusting and lateral movements, as well as by active licking.

Parents are often advised to check that their baby is no longer displaying the tongue-thrust reflex before beginning complementary feeding, but since it has usually disappeared by 6 months (which is when the introduction of solid foods is recommended), this is an unnecessary precaution in most cases. It may, however, be relevant for babies whose development is atypical, in whom the reflex may persist for longer, offering them prolonged protection until they are ready to begin the transition to chewing solid foods (see page 131). It's also important to note that while the presence of the extrusion reflex in babies older than 6 months may be considered a reason not to embark on spoon feeding by an adult, the same does not apply to BLW, since the self-feeding baby is already in control of what goes into his mouth.

The gag reflex

Gagging and coughing occur fairly commonly in the early days of eating solid foods. They are both normal reflexes, which exist to prevent food or other objects from entering the airway and to help keep pieces of food from being swallowed before they have been sufficiently broken down by chewing. However, they are often incorrectly identified or, crucially, mistaken for choking. The different features of gagging, coughing, and choking are summarized in Table 1, on page 73.

The gag reflex involves the muscles of the jaw, larynx, and pharynx (throat), as well as upward peristaltic (wavelike) movements of the esophagus. It is generally triggered by the presence of food toward the back of the mouth, although in a very young baby, the trigger point may be as far forward as the tip of the tongue. When the reflex is activated, there is a combined, coordinated muscular contraction, which lowers the jaw, raises the back of the tongue, closes off the airway, and pushes the food forward in a retching movement.[19] Provided the baby is in an upright position the food will be either pushed out of his mouth or returned to the gums for more chewing. Occasionally, the reflex will result in a small vomit but in many cases the baby will carry on eating as if nothing has happened.

Babies can gag on strips and small pieces of food but they can also gag on purees. Parental reports and clinical observations suggest that gagging episodes triggered by a strip of food are shorter and less distressing than those involving small pieces and purees because the baby can simply pull the strip out of his mouth. This ability to manage gagging not only helps babies learn safe eating techniques but also increases their confidence. Over time, they will discover other methods of dealing with troublesome food, first pushing it out with their tongue, then removing it from their mouth with their fingers, and eventually—as toddlers—learning to purposefully spit out anything they don't like or can't break down sufficiently.

TABLE 1. GAGGING, COUGHING, AND CHOKING

	GAGGING	COUGHING	CHOKING
What it is	An innate reflex, present at birth. Common occurrence.	An innate reflex, present at birth. Fairly common occurrence.	Rare occurrence. Result of failure or bypassing of gag and cough reflexes and/or poorly coordinated closure of the larynx.
What it does	Pushes food that is not ready to be swallowed away from the oropharynx, toward the front of the mouth. Protects the airway and the esophagus.	Causes rapid expulsion of food or other object from the oropharynx/trachea, clearing the airway.	Food or other object lodges in the upper airway (oropharynx/larynx/trachea), blocking the passage of air in and out.
How it works	Back of tongue humps up and pharyngeal (throat) muscles contract in a forward movement.	Chest and throat muscles contract to force a blast of air from the lungs.	Airway is either completely blocked or severely narrowed. No (or almost no) air can get past the obstruction. Baby cannot breathe, so cannot cough.
What it looks and sounds like	Baby makes a retching movement, which may be soundless. Depending on skin tone, face may appear flushed or red. Eyes may water.	Baby makes a coughing sound—usually loud. Depending on skin tone, face may appear flushed or red. Eyes may water	Baby is silent or wheezing. Depending on skin tone, face may appear darkened, dusky or blue. Baby may appear frightened, wave arms, or clutch at throat
What you need to do	Ensure baby is in an upright position. Observe quietly and provide reassurance. Once over, baby carries on eating/chewing.	Ensure baby is in an upright position. Observe quietly and provide reassurance. Once over, baby carries on eating.	Act fast. Call for help. Begin approved first aid measures to clear the obstruction.

I sought help with feeding when my Owen turned 9 months because he seemed to gag on purees and have a strong reaction to foods. With coaching we were able to transition away from purees and spoon feeding to table foods. The changeover was amazingly quick, and Owen now eats what we eat.

Megan, mother of Owen, 10 months

Gagging in children with feeding challenges

In a baby with a food aversion, even the sight or smell of food, or its texture when touched, can be enough to cause gagging, and he may show distress. Over time, and with repeated exposure and practice, the reflex becomes desensitized, so that he will eventually gag only if anything gets close to his airway. Similarly, babies and children who have underlying sensory processing issues often have an oversensitive gag reflex—indeed, this may be the first sign that such a problem exists. Selecting foods in the early weeks that are less likely to trigger the reflex—like a food strip that won't break—will help lessen the risk of the baby's developing negative associations with food, while allowing gradual desensitization.

The cough reflex

The cough reflex is triggered farther back in a baby's mouth than the gag reflex and occurs when mucus, liquid, or an object or piece of food is at the level of the vocal folds and directly threatening the airway. Coughing involves the muscles of the chest, which contract to create a blast of air from the lungs, propelling the potential obstruction forward. While gagging is usually quiet, coughing is always noisy—although this distinction is blurred when the two occur together. Both gagging and coughing may be accompanied by crying, and both tend to increase blood flow to the face, giving the baby a flushed appearance. In paler skin this will show as redness but the change may be less obvious in darker skin tones. It's also common for the baby's eyes to water and for them to spit or dribble saliva. As with gagging, a baby who is coughing will usually be able to clear the obstruction unaided, provided he is in an upright position.

Choking

Choking describes a situation where the reflexes of gagging and coughing have failed to clear the obstruction or been bypassed. A baby whose airway is completely blocked will be silent because no air can get in or out, while a partial blockage may allow the escape of some air, leading to a wheezing sound. Because he is unable to breathe the baby's face will tend to lose color, looking gray, dusky, or blue (also likely to be less apparent in darker complexions), and he may appear frightened. A baby who is choking needs urgent assistance.

Research shows there is no difference in the frequency or occurrence of choking between babies who are introduced to solid foods using BLW and those who are spoon fed.[20] However, parents and others caring for babies with neurodevelopmental challenges, muscular weakness, or a limited range of movement need to pay special attention to the shape, size, and texture of foods offered, since these babies may initially have more difficulty maneuvering them than their typically developing peers. For all babies, frequent opportunities to explore food and to practice and hone their feeding skills on a large variety of differently sized, shaped, and textured foods will help them to become efficient and safe eaters.

Skills for managing solid foods

These are the skills that a baby needs to master in order to feed himself safely and independently with solid foods. In babies whose development is typical, these skills usually appear between 6 and 12 months. However, babies with a medical or developmental disorder that affects their feeding may not acquire them until significantly later.

- sufficient head and neck control to hold his head upright without tiring
- sufficient balance and postural stability to maintain a sitting position with minimal support (e.g., in a chair) without falling to the side or slumping forward
- the ability to reach out accurately toward things that interest him (eye-hand coordination)
- fine motor skills, beginning with a raking movement (made by extending one or more fingers and then drawing them back) and palmar grasp, progressing to a pincer grasp, using thumb and forefinger
- the ability to bring his hand to his mouth purposefully
- the ability to open his mouth to accommodate a bite of food, and, over time, to grade the degree of opening
- the ability to close his lips to facilitate a swallow
- the ability to move food from the center of his mouth to the chewing surfaces of his gums and teeth
- dissociation of his tongue, lips, and jaw, so that they can move independently as well as together

Developing advanced eating skills

From birth, babies naturally eat and drink using just their mouth and their hands. However, most parents want their children to follow the accepted practices of their culture and learn to do the same as those around them. So, utensils of some sort are likely to feature once solid foods are introduced, along with bowls, plates, and cups.

Utensils

Not every culture employs utensils for eating—and those that do tend to use items that are traditional within that nation or social group. In the developed world, for young children, that usually means spoons, forks, and/or chopsticks.

It's worth noting that the utensils we most often associate with babies, namely spoons, have more to do with allowing an adult to control the child's eating than with the needs of the baby himself. Unfortunately, as a result of the trend toward giving solid foods to younger and younger babies, spoon feeding small children became the norm (see "The phenomenon of spoon feeding," page 19). Indeed, the majority of the academic and professional discourse on infant feeding puts great stress on the "skill" of taking food off a spoon, even implying that it is an integral part of "natural" development. In fact, it is a learned skill that most babies do not need to acquire until they are ready to begin using a spoon to feed themselves.

Typically developing babies of 6 months can hold a spoon and take it to their mouth. If it is pre-loaded, they can usually get at least some of the food from it, although they will often turn it upside down in the process. This is the natural consequence of the way in which they bring their hand to their mouth. Some babies can dip a spoon into soft food from around 8 months, but scooping up the food and turning the wrist so as to keep the bowl of the spoon upright is a much more complex skill that most don't master until they are around 12 months or older. Forks tend to be easier to manage: Most 6-month-olds can take food from a small pre-loaded fork without difficulty, and some will be able to spear a piece of food with a fork by about 10 months. This is a more logical progression for a baby who is used to being offered pieces of food as opposed to purees and mashes. A single chopstick can also be used to spear food, although managing a pair of chopsticks is rare before 15 months at the earliest.

The key to helping babies use utensils for themselves is for other family members to model this behavior during shared mealtimes and to encourage experimentation without any expectations of success. From 6 months, and especially from around 9 months, babies are very aware of the actions of others and determined to mimic them. They also enjoy mastering new skills, but refinement takes time. Initially, they will tend to be distracted or frustrated by their efforts at using utensils, and it may be many months before they no longer revert to using their hands and fingers, especially for more challenging foods.

Cups

Cup drinking is possible from a very young age. Most pre-term babies can take small amounts by cup, using a lapping action, before full breastfeeding is possible. However, adult-style drinking is a different skill, which babies will need when they move on from breast- or bottle feeding. It requires an element of jaw stability, strength in the cheek muscles, and coordination of sucking, swallowing, and breathing. The upper lip must come down and forward to meet the cup while the lower lip tenses to provide stability; this requires the two lips to work together, but separately from the tongue and jaw. The cheeks then need to contract, creating a partial vacuum to draw the liquid in and channel it back for swallowing. Many babies of 6 months have these skills—even those who are experiencing feeding difficulties—they just need to refine them, which takes practice.

Many 6-month-olds can hold a cup independently, using two hands (or one hand for very small cups), and they quickly discover how to tip it just the right amount. Picking up the cup and replacing it on the tray or table without knocking it over is a more complex skill, which some will manage by around 10 months. Covered cups with a valve (whether sippy cups or 360) are not recommended by speech and language therapists and orthodontists, since they encourage inappropriate use of the oral muscles (see page 22). In particular, they promote an immature suckling action, using the tongue. An open cup is ideal, preferably one the size of a shot glass, since a narrow circumference is a more effective and leak-free fit for a baby's mouth.

It is sometimes suggested that it is best to start with a very small amount of liquid in the cup, to reduce the likelihood of spills. However, although it may feel counterintuitive, filling a small cup at least half full can make it easier for a novice drinker to manage alone, because there is less need to tilt it. This allows the baby to focus on the skill of drinking rather than on controlling the degree of slant. It also prevents him from having to tip his head backward, which can interfere with his balance as well as make it more difficult for him to close his airway and swallow safely.

Straws

Straw drinking is a useful skill for all babies to acquire—not only because it enables practice at movements needed for clear speech but because it makes drinking while traveling easier and less messy. Using a straw requires similar control and technique to using a cup but with exaggerated lip rounding and use of the cheek muscles and with retraction of the tongue. The tip of the straw should rest between the lips; it should not extend into the mouth or lie on the surface of the tongue. Straws that do not have a valve are preferable for teaching babies the correct technique.

Most babies can learn to drink independently from a straw between 6 and 9 months of age. The trick is to persuade them to keep sucking, without releasing the vacuum, until they get the liquid into their mouth. It can be helpful to show them what is supposed to happen by placing a pre-filled pipette or straw between their lips and releasing a small amount of liquid every time they suck. Once they understand the process, the next challenge is for them to learn to control their suck, so as not to overfill their mouth and have liquid spilling out. The shorter the straw, the easier this will be.

In typically developing babies, the feeding skills described in this chapter tend to emerge in parallel, in much the same order, and within a well-defined age range. However, they may appear considerably later, and mature more gradually, in babies whose development is delayed or who are unable to practice the necessary movements because of anatomical or functional differences. This will be exacerbated if the baby is not provided with frequent opportunities for copying and repetition, or if he is not exposed to real food that will stimulate interest and experimentation. The next chapter looks at the sorts of obstacles, faced by babies whose development does not follow the usual pathways, that can combine to make the transition to solid food especially challenging.

REWEY'S STORY

Jill's account

REWEY'S HISTORY

Rewey is her parents' second child. She has an older brother who has a history of speech and sensory issues and a diagnosis of apraxia, which affects voluntary movements. Soon after birth, Rewey was noted to have a shortened muscle on one side of her neck (torticollis) and delayed motor development, both of which affected her ability to feed effectively, and for which she began receiving physical therapy. She was also diagnosed with severe gastroesophageal reflux (GER). A combination of the torticollis, which restricted her head movements, and the fact that the reflux prevented her from spending time on her tummy meant that Rewey began to show signs of a flattening of the skull bones on one side of her head (plagiocephaly). In order to resolve this, she wore a helmet for four months until her head shape improved and she was able to have more tummy time. At 7 months, she began treatment with medication to decrease the production of stomach acid. Attempts to wean her off this medication at 12 months were unsuccessful, and she eventually stopped needing it at 15.5 months.

Rewey was exclusively breastfed until 6 months, when her mom began to introduce formula. This was prompted partly by her mom's return to work and partly to make sure Rewey was getting enough milk, since they had begun a program of sleep training. At the same time, she introduced some spoon-fed solid foods, like oatmeal, sweet potato, apple, and pears, most of which she couldn't even get into Rewey's mouth, as she would shake her head no. If any did make it into her mouth, she would immediately push it out with her tongue.

I met Rewey when she was 6.5 months old, as part of a joint developmental screening session with a physical therapist, which was held virtually. At that time, she had evidence of some delay in her gross motor development, as well as persistent torticollis, and she did not tolerate lying on her tummy because of discomfort from the reflux. She was spitting up fifteen to twenty times a day, but—remarkably—was managing to gain weight well. Following the screening, I recommended feeding therapy and offered to take her case. I also referred her for an assessment by a dietitian and advised that she continue with physical therapy.

REWEY'S FEEDING THERAPY INTERVENTION AND PROGRESS

Rewey's feeding therapy began at 8 months, alongside the physical therapy and support from a dietitian to ensure adequate intake of calories and micronutrients. Progress was slow, as Rewey would cry when put in her high chair, which her brother couldn't tolerate. He would get extremely upset and scream, making mealtimes very complicated for the family. At the time, Rewey's father was out of the country for an extended period for work, and his early return home was arranged so that he could provide additional support during this stressful period.

We started by offering Rewey spoons pre-loaded with mashed table foods (such as avocado or sweet potato), starter food strips (such as a raw carrot strip), and a silicone feeder filled with a commercial puree. Mostly, she was happy to explore the food but less interested in eating it. For example, she would grasp a pre-loaded spoon or feeder but might put the handle in her mouth rather than the end containing the food. She was, however, willing to put her finger into food mashes and then bring it to her mouth. It quickly became clear that she preferred big foods that allowed her more control and didn't break apart, like steak strips and rib bones. She gagged occasionally and dropped lots of food on the floor as well as getting it in her hair, which was frustrating for her mom.

Rewey's frequent reflux and episodes of vomiting caused her to develop an aversion to the bottle. Unfortunately, when she was teething, she was sometimes disinterested in solid foods as well. Her parents were initially thickening her formula feeds with oatmeal, which appeared to be causing constipation. Guided by the dietitian, they switched the oatmeal for purees. This, together with shorter, more frequent feedings and an emphasis on responsive feeding and the need to follow Rewey's cues, all helped to decrease her aversion to being fed by bottle. At around the same time, I suggested that Rewey switch to a chair with an adjustable footrest, so that her eating position was more stable. She initially resisted this, so feeding sessions often had to begin on mom's lap (something that is occasionally still necessary). However, a better feeding position, combined with a baby-led approach that allowed Rewey to control what and how much went into her mouth, had a positive and profound impact on her eating skills.

From 9 to 12 months, Rewey became happier to sit in her chair and was beginning to feed herself mashes, like yogurt mixed with ground peanuts, from her tray. She began to gnaw on large foods, such as peeled kiwi and peach, and to take bites from soft solid strips, like avocado. She could eat pieces of scrambled egg mixed with avocado, or combined foods (for example, black beans with rice) with her fingers. She slowly began to extend the amount of time she would spend in her high chair and to pick up and eat food pieces using a pincer grasp. She was also able to drink slightly thinned purees from an open cup, with assistance, and to use a straw independently. She continued to have bottles of formula thickened with purees to help with the vomiting. However, they seemed to be interfering with her appetite, so the dietitian worked with Rewey's mom to reduce the amount of puree in each bottle.

At the time of writing, Rewey is 14 months old and currently eats a wide variety of differently shaped, sized, and textured table foods. She has been slightly more resistant to sitting in her chair since she began walking independently and discovering other activities, and she tends to be inconsistent in her interest in table foods and self-feeding. This appears to be related to how she is feeling emotionally and physically, as well as to the stress levels within the home when her brother is having a hard time. Overall, though, she is adjusting well to family meals and beginning to enjoy the business of eating.

DISCUSSION

Rewey's progress has been quite remarkable. In just six months she has gone from being 100 percent spoon fed with jarred baby foods, which she would often refuse, to independent self-feeding of strips, large foods, and pieces of table foods. Looking back, most of her problems appear to have stemmed from her reflux. This was clearly causing her a lot of pain, even with the medication. She seemed to be able to cope better if she could pace her eating—and she could only really do this when she was in control of what was happening. Adapted BLW gave her that control. It also gave her the opportunity to practice movements that aren't required when a baby is spoon fed, helping to improve her motor strength and coordination. The combination of physical therapy and fine motor practice that she received during these six months resulted in resolved torticollis and independent walking by the age of 13 months, with no evidence of residual motor delay.

Rewey's mom's perspective

When you are expecting your second child, the number of times you hear, "Oh, just wait . . . every kid is different" can become nauseating. I thought to myself: *I've done this already. I must know what I'm doing.*

When our daughter started choking on her vomit in her hospital bassinet twenty-four hours after she was born, I realized I was wrong. Her reflux started literally at birth and it was not anything I was prepared for or had any experience with. I only recall our son throwing up once during the infant stage, but for the first four to five months of her life Rewey threw up constantly. This was accompanied by screaming and refusal to be put down, which probably contributed to her motor delay. So many people assured me that starting solids would "make the reflux much better," so I was hopeful.

I eagerly waited for our pediatrician to clear Rewey to eat solids, and once she did I jumped right in . . . only to hit a wall. Every time I would offer her any sort of food from a spoon, she would shake her head no and scream in protest. I was encouraged by the pediatrician to "keep trying," so this went on for quite a while. I never once was successfully able to get her to take any purees, rice cereal, oatmeal, etc., from me during that time. Initially, I wasn't aware that feeding therapy was an option, but I quickly had Rewey evaluated once I knew it was available. I think she threw up eleven times in the hour-long virtual evaluation.

When we started working with Jill, I felt really intimidated by the concepts she was trying to implement with our daughter. I had heard of baby-led weaning when our son was little, but it seemed so out of reach. It felt like I needed to do mounds of research on the topic in order to be successful. And I also thought giving huge chunks of food to babies with no teeth sounded like a recipe for disaster. I remember when Jill first suggested I give Rewey large pieces of food to practice jaw movement, I honestly considered just quitting the whole process. I was so nervous that I was putting her at risk because those first few sessions were mostly about letting her work her jaw on foods that would not break off, which meant she still was not really "eating anything."

The thought of my daughter gnawing on a strip of steak seemed absolutely crazy to me and I did not understand how that would help her to accept purees from me off a spoon, but it was amazing to see how much Rewey's face lit up when I handed her that strip of steak and let her just gum it! She was finally getting to taste something flavorful—and the key was that it was on her terms. I never realized it was the reflux that had caused her to have such an aversion to eating. Anytime I would try to feed her myself, there was an outright refusal—it caused her so much discomfort and stress that she wanted to be in charge.

I was candidly shocked at how many tips and tricks Jill was able to give us to get Rewey eating—all by letting her feed herself. I was appreciative of how it was a gradual process. We started with letting her gnaw on strips, then moved to picking up mushed foods, then eating pieces of real food. It never ceases to amaze me to watch her hold and eat an entire kiwi all by herself! At 14 months old, she is better at feeding herself than my almost 4-year-old! I wish we had used this approach with our older child because it has been so easy.

4
.....

Identifying Babies at Risk for Feeding Challenges

Feeding difficulties are a common feature of infancy and the toddler years,[1] but they are considerably more likely in children whose development follows an atypical path or who have physical or medical anomalies. Feeding difficulties in infancy can not only affect health and well-being during babyhood but may also track into childhood and even adulthood. Early identification of potential—as well as actual—problems, and timely and appropriate intervention are therefore extremely important.

Some feeding difficulties stem directly from anatomical differences, while others arise from medical or surgical treatments or traumatic eating experiences. Some are the result of a simple lack of oral feeding in the early weeks and months. This chapter explains the importance of early intervention to reduce the long-term effects of these types of challenge.

Innate feeding challenges

There are many different medical conditions and syndromes that will likely be associated with feeding difficulties. Some of these will be known at birth, while others will manifest later. In addition to the challenges presented by the diagnosis, these babies are also at risk of developing an aversion to feeding, owing to the types of treatment they may be required to undergo. These issues are discussed on page 95.

Neuromotor and developmental issues

Babies who have neuromotor and developmental difficulties include those with an identified syndrome, such as Noonan syndrome, Down syndrome, Williams syndrome, or Prader-Willi syndrome. These infants may face challenges with movement (both muscular and neurological in origin) as well as overall developmental delay, all of which will impact their gross motor and fine motor foundational skills. Other babies that may fall into this category include pre-term infants, especially those born very early, such as Addie (see Addie's story, page 113)[2]; babies with a cerebral birth injury or complicated birth history; and those with other, specific neuromuscular issues.

All babies who have neuromotor and/or developmental issues are likely to have difficulties with posture, stability when sitting, and hand-to-mouth movements, which will require individualized support for them to be able to self-feed. This can delay the timeline in which they may begin self-feeding and affect how they learn to self-feed compared with their neurotypical peers. They may also face challenges with coordination of breathing and swallowing, eye-hand coordination, tongue movement, chewing, and/or swallowing.[3] Babies with Down syndrome, for example, tend to have particular difficulty with refined tongue movements and swallowing.[4]

Babies with visual impairment also fall into this group; however, their challenges are slightly different. While parents may wonder how a child with impaired vision can feed herself, being spoon fed will likely be the more stressful option for a baby who has visual difficulties. This is partly because of the difficulty of anticipating the arrival of the spoon and the need to coordinate her movements with those of her caregiver, and partly because her reliance on touch will be greater than for a baby with full vision. It is easy for feeding to feel intrusive to a child who has no means of identifying what is happening; self-feeding may be a better way to build confidence.

> As a former labor and delivery nurse, I was committed to breastfeeding my baby and the natural evolution of that seemed to be baby-led weaning. When I found out my daughter would have Down syndrome, I wasn't sure if either of those things would be possible.
>
> Ella Gray Cullen, mom of Julia Grace, 5 years

Cardio-respiratory compromise

Difficulties in breathing, disordered or weak heart function, and issues connected with blood circulation or the blood's ability to carry oxygen can all lead to feeding difficulties. This may be because breathing is rapid or labored, making coordination of sucking (or biting and chewing), swallowing, and breathing difficult, or it can simply be that the effort required is tiring. A baby who lacks the stamina for sustained feeding may need to rely on tube feedings for a prolonged period, either as her sole mode of feeding or as a supportive measure. However, as she gains in strength and ability, the more opportunity she has to control the manner and speed of her eating, the easier the process will be and the safer she will feel.

Anatomical and/or structural issues

Babies who are born with structural anomalies of the head, face, and/or neck commonly face feeding challenges. Conditions such as tracheoesophageal fistula (an abnormal opening between the trachea and the esophagus), laryngeal cleft (an opening connecting the larynx and the esophagus), or laryngomalacia (low muscle tone in the larynx) tend to impede swallowing and the coordination of swallowing and breathing. When babies have structural anomalies that impact respiration, they will always choose breathing in preference to eating, so food refusal is common.

Babies with cleft lip and palate commonly struggle with milk feeding, owing to difficulties in achieving a seal with their lips, and creating the partial vacuum needed to extract milk. They may also find chewing and swallowing challenging. They may require modifications to their food, such as thickening of liquids and softening of solid foods to make them easier to break down. They also face the prospect of multiple surgeries and unpleasant or painful treatments.

In recent years there has been a big increase in the diagnosis of tethered oral tissues (TOTs), such as tongue and lip ties. These tend to cause difficulties with breast- or bottle feeding but may affect the baby's ability to manage solid foods as well. This is especially true of a tongue-tie, in which the restrictive lingual frenulum prevents the elevation of the tongue necessary for safe swallowing or hampers its sideways movement (lateralization) and impedes the movement of food to the gums for chewing (see Luke's story, page 26). Restrictions that impact the baby's ability to chew sufficiently or manage a bolus of food in her mouth can lead to fatigue and frustration, and result in a preference for soft foods that require little chewing. Tongue-ties and other TOTs are generally easy to treat; the earlier they are diagnosed, the quicker this can happen and the less impact there will be on feeding.

Digestive issues and food intolerances

Babies who have digestive problems, such as gastroesophageal reflux (GER) or gastroesophageal reflux disease (GERD), may struggle with transitioning to solid foods. Chronic reflux commonly leads the baby to associate feeding with an unpleasant taste, pain and/or vomiting, or the burning sensation that accompanies aspiration of stomach contents into the lungs. Babies with as yet unidentified allergies or intolerances to certain foods (for example, dairy or wheat) may make similar associations if they experience mild or severe discomfort when they eat trigger foods—possibly at every mealtime. Some babies appear to have an increased sensitivity to pain in the stomach and intestines (and other internal organs), known as visceral hyperalgesia. In many cases this seems to follow an illness or injury but the exact cause is unclear. These babies often appear to be in constant discomfort, which is made worse by eating.

Some babies who have had a negative gut-related (or "interoceptive") experience are able to connect this with certain foods, which they will try to avoid—something they are more likely to be able to do if foods are presented individually rather than as combined dishes. Others decide that all food must be avoided. They may agree to eat a bare minimum of solid food (often referred to as "self-limiting"), relying instead on human milk or infant formula as their primary nutrition well past the time that they should be enjoying a varied diet.

A warning sign exhibited by some very young babies with digestive issues is that they will breast- or bottle feed only when sleeping. Then, when solid foods are first introduced, they avoid or refuse foods to which they are later discovered to be intolerant or allergic. For example, a baby who consistently refuses to eat foods that contain gluten may turn out to have a diagnosis of celiac disease. Babies vary in the signs they display, but behaviors that suggest a desire to avoid food always warrant investigation.

Sensory issues

Some babies have issues related to the taste, odor, temperature, and/or texture of particular foods or groups of foods, often for reasons that are not obvious to their parents. For example, they may be wary of foods that they have found to be unreliable, such as fruits that can be either sweet or tart, or that vary in texture depending on their ripeness. The anxiety induced by these features is likely to make them cautious about trying anything new or eating something that has taken them by surprise in the past. They may cling to snack foods, whose texture and flavor are more constant and predictable. They may gag or vomit on chunks of food or more textured purees, or even at the sight, smell, or feel of certain foods. They may cry when placed in the high chair or refuse to engage with the food, turning away from it or throwing it on the floor. They may splay their fingers while eating, or want their hands wiped frequently. As they get older they may agree to eat only specifically colored or textured food, only very bland foods, or only certain brands of commercially made food—or they may simply display a lack of appetite or a general disinterest in food. Babies who restrict their intake in this way are at increased risk of insufficient weight gain and micronutrient deficiencies.

Strong sensory responses and underresponsiveness to foods have both been found to be connected with disorders that affect muscle tone,[5] whether unusually high (hypertonia) or low (hypotonia). This can mean that the baby gets too much or too little feedback from the touch receptors inside her mouth, prompting her to take excessively large bites or to overstuff her mouth. Exaggerated sensory responses may also indicate an undiagnosed food intolerance or allergy, which should always be investigated as a possible explanation. Alternatively, they may be linked to underlying difficulties in interpreting or responding to sensory information. These may extend to textures, colors, and smells beyond the arena of food, manifesting as a reluctance to touch certain fabrics or play materials, or an aversion to loud sounds. Behaviors such as these are sometimes seen in older children who have a diagnosis of autism. If sensory issues are evident without an apparent underlying cause, it may be appropriate to confer with an occupational therapist and/or developmental pediatrician. A full assessment of the child's sensory system will determine whether there is an underlying medical or behavioral cause and may lead to a meaningful diagnosis.

Trauma-induced feeding aversion

Babies who experience trauma can develop an aversion to feeding. While some types of trauma are preventable, others are an unavoidable part of the complicated care required by babies who have medical or developmental disorders. Trauma-induced feeding issues may present with behaviors similar to those seen in babies who have sensory or interoceptive issues, namely refusal to eat certain (or all) foods, self-limiting intake, and crying while eating or when placed in a high chair. The baby may also show a preference for liquids or pureed foods over those that require chewing or spend long periods playing with food in order to avoid eating. Behaviors such as throwing food, pushing the food or spoon away, kicking and arm waving, and gagging or vomiting in response to food are also common.

Pain or discomfort associated with feeding—for example, difficulty in swallowing (dysphagia), a burning sensation caused by reflux or aspiration, gut pain from an allergic reaction or hypersensitivity of the nerves in the stomach, or disruption to breathing resulting from inhalation of food via a cleft—can have huge ramifications for infants, especially when it occurs repeatedly. Such experiences can quickly lead to an aversion to food or to being fed—as with Henry (see page 44). Unfortunately, illnesses such as celiac disease and eosinophilic esophagitis (EoE) are often not formally diagnosed until the toddler years, allowing unpleasant associations with food to build up over many months. Without understanding how or why, the baby rightly concludes that eating is going to cause her distress, so she tries to avoid it at all costs. An added complication is that anxiety itself can lead to a loss of appetite, giving the baby an additional reason to refuse food.[6]

Extremely pre-term infants and those with a complicated medical history can develop a different type of feeding aversion. These babies often have to undergo frequent, intrusive, and unpleasant medical interventions, particularly to their mouth and face, such as suctioning, nasogastric tube placement, or insertion of a breathing tube (intubation). Experiences such as these can lead the baby to respond fearfully when anyone or anything approaches her face, and especially her mouth or nose. Her initial encounters with food and feeding may also be painful, unpleasant, and anxiety-provoking. Add to this the likelihood of prolonged periods of hospitalization, with some degree of separation from parents and the necessity for care to be provided by multiple strangers, and it's easy to see how feeding difficulties can arise.

A fear of eating or being fed can follow a traumatic choking episode. Choking is especially likely to happen if the feeding situation is unsafe—for example, if the baby is leaning back or slumped, or if she has been given food of a size or consistency that she is unable to manage. In some cases, the alarmed response of a caregiver is enough to make the baby fearful and anxious thereafter, even if the event itself was not life-threatening. Fear of eating can also be the result of repeated instances of overfeeding. This may have been forceful, in which case the infant is likely to be afraid of the feeding situation, or it may have been coercive or achieved via a gavage tube, such that the baby was unable to indicate satiety and so suffered the pain of a distended stomach. If the overfeeding resulted in vomiting or choking, this will have exacerbated the trauma.

Fear of food, of eating, or of being fed, especially as the result of one or more vomiting or choking episodes linked to a specific food, often manifests as a refusal to taste, or take a bite of, the same food when it is offered again for fear that the same thing will happen. It can also lead to the development of what is sometimes referred to as "conditioned dysphagia,"[7] which is difficulty in swallowing that doesn't have an underlying medical cause. This can present as refusal to swallow certain foods. Wariness of tasting, biting, or swallowing may extend to other foods or textures that the child perceives as similar, and that therefore trigger the same anxiety response.

Attempts to overfeed a child or force them to eat are rarely malicious. They can be the result of genuine parental (or professional) concerns over food intake, prompted by any of the scenarios described above. They can also be triggered by a family history of picky eating, or a situation where lack of food is, or was previously, a reality. Similarly, many parents of children who have feeding difficulties understandably carry a lot of anxiety, which can easily be transmitted to the baby. Sensitive and careful discussion between the family and feeding professionals may help to untangle the background to the situation and the emotions involved, and enable a more responsive feeding approach.

> As I see it, the only way through mealtime worry is to let children go at their own pace and be partners in the process.
>
> Marsha Dunn Klein, occupational therapist and founder of the Get Permission Institute

Babies who are—or have been—tube fed

Babies who have a long history of gavage feedings, either via a nasogastric tube (passed through the nose) or through a gastrostomy tube (inserted through the skin of the abdomen) are another group at risk for feeding difficulties when they transition to oral feeding. Many have a complicated history, in which their nutritional needs are calculated for them and their hunger and satiety cues largely ignored. This is especially true where feeding is continuous rather than in separately measured bolus amounts. They may experience overfeeding and frequent vomiting, as well as extended dependence on formulas. They may lack sufficient oral experience to enable them to connect the sensation of a full stomach with the action of feeding. And they will rarely have had any opportunity to look at, smell, touch, or taste the food they are "eating." This can make the transition to solid foods extremely challenging.

Our youngest child was diagnosed with Noonan Syndrome, along with associated medical complexities, and had a long stay in the NICU. He was discharged on a nasogastric tube and each feeding was a challenge. The self-feeding approach was scary at first but we quickly saw the benefits. Our son is now quite the foodie and enjoys every second of mealtime!

Margie and Mike, parents of Luke, 7 years

It is easy to see how, faced with challenges such as these, parents and babies can quickly come to dread mealtimes. Feeding interventions that use a responsive feeding approach, where there is no pressure to eat large volumes or particular foods, can provide a positive way forward. Adapted baby-led weaning takes this thinking one step further, allocating control and decision-making to the child, thereby removing the sense of being "done to" and replacing it with true autonomy.

Anticipating and preventing feeding difficulties

Anticipation and prevention—or, at least, early detection—of feeding difficulties is important, not just because such problems make eating and drinking challenging but because they carry significant risks in both the short and long term. Many of these can be minimized if the problem is identified promptly and the appropriate treatment, therapy or management instituted.

Swallowing difficulties

Dysphagia, or difficulty swallowing, is a key factor in the feeding difficulties faced by many babies. It can be the result of
structural anomalies of the mouth or throat, or low muscle
tone. It is also a feature of certain syndromes and can accom-
pany other, more general neuromotor difficulties. For some
babies, swallowing issues present a real risk of choking and
aspiration (see Theodora's story, page 235). Swallowing is a
complex process involving many different structures of the
mouth and throat; accurate identification of the nature of the
problem is paramount.

If a baby appears to be having difficulty swallowing, or there
are signs that liquid is spilling over into her airway, those treat-
ing her will want to visualize how the muscles of her mouth
and throat function during a swallow. There are two ways in
which this can be done. The first is a videofluoroscopic swallowing study (VFSS), or modified barium swallow, which is a
moving X-ray image using a radiopaque feed. The second, a
fiberoptic endoscopic evaluation of swallowing (FEES), uses a
thin, flexible instrument to see inside the baby's throat. A FEES
is often preferred for a baby or young child because it avoids
the use of X-rays, can be done in an office or clinic, and may
be used to assess swallowing during both breast- and bottle
feeding. However, because the endoscope is passed via the
baby's nose, the oral part of the swallow cannot be observed.

Where food or liquid is seen to enter the larynx during swallowing, the results of the VFSS or FEES will help determine a
suitable degree of viscosity for the baby's foods and drinks.
Milk feeds and other fluids can then be thickened accordingly,

and solid foods can be chosen to match the baby's abilities (see Henry's story, page 44). The International Dysphagia Diet Standardisation Initiative (IDDSI) has created a globally recognized framework, which allows descriptions of the consistency of what the baby should be offered to be universally understood and easily followed.[8] Those caring for babies who are known or suspected to aspirate while drinking need to adhere closely to the liquid specifications, to ensure the baby's safety.

While some swallowing difficulties may resolve spontaneously, most babies with dysphagia will need to be followed closely by a medical and therapeutic team to assist in selecting therapy techniques, appropriate food textures, sizes and shapes, and liquid viscosity to ensure safety in swallowing. The decision to transition to thinner liquids or a more complex food texture will usually be made only after a repeat VFSS or FEES confirms that there has been an improvement in the baby's swallowing skills.

> Sam was born at 26 weeks. On day 5 he had emergency surgery to remove a section of his intestine. He spent 151 days in the NICU. Then, when he came home, we discovered that he was aspirating when taking his bottle. He was on thickened feeds for the next 14 months, during which time he started solids with self-feeding. At 20 months (17 adjusted), his jaw and mouth are so strong that not only can he bite and pull strong enough to handle any food, but he is doing incredibly well with his speech as well.
>
> Ben and Maureen, parents of Sam,
> born at 26 weeks' gestation

Longer-term risks

A failure to diagnose feeding difficulties promptly, and to devise and implement a plan to manage them, can impact the baby's well-being and success with eating longer than need be the case. Four risks stand out. The first is that the baby's diet may consist of a very limited range of foods—for example, only fruit, or white foods, or ultra-processed snack foods. This means she can easily lack important nutrients, putting her at risk of poor weight gain and micronutrient deficiencies. Second, the baby may get stuck on a diet of purees, leading to problems with chewing different textures in later childhood.[9] A super-soft diet can also lead to suboptimal growth of the facial bones and muscles,[10] which may be particularly important for babies whose facial anatomy is already affected by a physical anomaly. In addition, babies whose experience is primarily with pureed foods (many of which are similar in appearance) will have only a limited reference list of "real" foods that they recognize. When, as toddlers, they start to move away from purees at just the same time as the typical wariness toward new foods (neophobia) kicks in, they may begin to refuse foods they previously accepted, just because they look different. This can mean that their diet becomes even more limited.

A third risk is that babies with an undiagnosed disorder (such as reflux or an allergy) are dismissed as "difficult feeders," or treated for behavioral problems, when in fact they are simply responding to what they are experiencing. Such misdirected management is likely to make the problem worse, not better. Finally, there is the risk that the stress experienced by caregivers faced with a child with feeding challenges will lead to poor reading of the baby's cues. This may mean that opportunities for feeding are missed. Alternatively, if there is concern over inadequate weight gain, it may result in force-feeding or pushing of large volumes of food. In extreme cases it can lead to a serious breakdown of the parent–child relationship, when what should be a mutually enjoyable and nurturing experience becomes filled with fear, pain, frustration, and guilt.

For all these reasons, it's crucial that feeding difficulties are anticipated, detected, assessed, and diagnosed as early as possible, so that an appropriately tailored therapeutic approach can be put in place. Ideally, this process should begin at birth.

Optimizing feeding in the first six months

Breastfeeding is the optimal way for newborn babies to feed.[11] It supports overall health and growth as well as optimizing nutrition, immune function, and facial shaping. It has also been found to enhance social and cognitive development. Exclusive breastfeeding is recommended by the World Health Organization for all babies for the first six months of life, with continued breastfeeding alongside complementary foods until the second birthday or beyond.[12] Babies with a medical diagnosis, who are at increased risk for health and developmental challenges, stand to benefit significantly from being breastfed—not only in terms of the active constituents of human milk but via the act of breastfeeding itself. This is because, through the frequent activation of specific facial muscles, breastfeeding provides a built-in oral motor exercise program, optimizing tongue movements, the shaping of the palate, and the space available for teeth to erupt. These aspects of physical growth are especially pertinent for babies whose facial structure and function are, or are likely to become, compromised.

Initial difficulties with breast- and/or bottle feeding can be a red flag for future feeding difficulties, especially when transitioning to solid foods, so it's important that babies are helped to feed safely and effectively from the very beginning. Conditions such as torticollis (a twisting or sideways tilting of the neck, caused by a shortened muscle) and low muscle tone can seriously interfere with the baby's ability to drink enough milk. The involvement of a lactation consultant can be crucial for achieving effective breastfeeding, while early input from speech-language, occupational, and physical therapists will help to optimize the progress of all babies who have a difficult start.

Moving on to complementary feeding

The move to complementary feeding involves not only new flavors but also a diversification of textures, which require a series of oral movements different from those needed for breast- or bottle feeding. These movements develop spontaneously but they may be delayed or develop atypically in children who are coping with medical and/or developmental challenges.

For certain groups, feeding difficulties can be predicted based on the baby's diagnosis (for example, Down syndrome or Noonan syndrome). Other babies may have a history of difficulties with milk feedings in the first few months, such as refusing the breast or bottle, coughing or leaking milk from the mouth while feeding, self-limiting their intake, vomiting, being willing to feed only when drowsy or sleeping, or crying when placed in a feeding position. In these situations, it is essential that a qualified feeding therapist carry out a full structural and functional feeding assessment to enable early identification of atypical oral motor and feeding skills—such as abnormal sucking, limited tongue elevation, or an open-mouth resting posture—and formation of a plan to address them. This will likely take the form of a pre-feeding program of targeted exercises for the jaw, cheeks, tongue, and lips (see page 126), which will help to equip the baby with optimal foundational skills long before the introduction of solid foods.

Babies who have a medical diagnosis associated with feeding difficulties and developmental delay may have unusually low or increased muscle tone, or neurological issues, that affect their gross motor development. This will have an impact on the baby's ability to sit and self-feed safely when it comes time to transition to solid foods, in addition to anticipated difficulties with the manipulation and chewing of food. Input from a physical therapist will help the baby achieve optimal core strength and stability. This will enable an upright sitting posture and accurate reaching and grasping, which will ensure that solid foods can be introduced safely as close to 6 months as possible and aid success in self-feeding. A physical therapist will also be able to provide therapeutic interventions to facilitate good head control, stable sitting, and accurate hand-to-mouth movements and advise parents on, for example, appropriate positioning and use of tummy time (see page 123).

A lag in motor development may mean that the introduction of complementary foods needs to be delayed beyond 6 months. Human milk or infant formula will usually continue to provide adequate nutrition until self-feeding is possible but, if the wait will be a long one, or if there are concerns about weight gain or micronutrient deficiencies, collaboration with an experienced dietitian will help to ensure the baby maintains an adequate intake of calories and macro- and micronutrients until she is developmentally ready to move forward with solid foods. It is more important to allow a baby time to develop the necessary strength and coordination than to begin solid feeding at the officially recommended age.

Rationale for a baby-led approach for babies with feeding challenges

Baby-led weaning has been shown to have many benefits for typically developing babies. All of these are relevant to neurodiverse babies, as well as to those who have other feeding challenges or who are at risk of developing a feeding aversion. In some cases, these babies may have even more to gain from a baby-led approach than their typically developing peers. For example, given that feeding difficulties are known to feature strongly in the lives of children with Down syndrome, an intervention that can prevent such problems has the potential to change the outlook for a baby born with this condition.[13]

Eating with others is generally more enjoyable than eating alone—for babies as well as adults. Sharing family mealtimes facilitates the passing on of cultural eating habits[14] and encourages the development of language.[15] It's also a great way for children to learn how to tackle foods presented in different ways, use utensils, and absorb simple table manners. Sadly, it's easy for those who need support with eating to miss out on the chance to join others at the table, because of a mistaken view that they need one-on-one attention if they are to eat anything. A focus on self-feeding means that even the youngest baby can be part of family mealtimes, joining in conversations and learning social skills right from the start.

Babies develop skills in response to the opportunities presented by their environment. They instinctively want to reach out and grab objects and use their mouth to explore them, and they are motivated to do the same with food. Indeed, food offers sensations and experiences that are unique and complex—it's the ultimate educational toy! Self-feeding using the hands facilitates the development of strong posture, gross and fine movements, and oral skills, as well as self-esteem and confidence, all of which can be difficult to achieve for babies whose opportunities for independent action are few.

Healthy food provides a foundation for optimal growth and development and the avoidance of illness. Allowing babies to decide what to eat from a selection of healthy food, to eat at their own pace, and to stop when their body tells them they've had enough helps to ensure optimal nourishment. Meanwhile, the gradualness of the changeover from milk to solid foods encouraged by ABLW, with human milk or infant formula featuring for longer than it tends to when feeding is parent-led, means that the infant is supported nutritionally while she develops the skills necessary for independent eating.

Keeping eating enjoyable and free from negative emotions, and enabling learning about a wide range of tastes and textures, assists the development of a positive relationship with food and helps to set the scene for a lifetime of healthy eating. But what makes an adapted form of baby-led weaning especially beneficial for babies with feeding challenges is its dual focus on self-feeding and foods that require chewing.

> ABLW works for babies who have all sorts of feeding difficulties: Whether it's transitioning from tube feeding to eating by mouth, learning to move their hands to their mouth, or effectively moving the food around for successful chewing and swallowing, this approach can help them achieve eating success.
>
> Karen Pryor, physical therapist and author

The case for textured foods

As discussed in chapter 1, historically it has been common for babies to be given purees as their first solid foods. This may be appropriate for very young infants, but the need for foods that are consistently smooth is questionable when solid foods are not introduced until around 6 months. At this age, or soon after, most babies are beginning to make chewing movements, so they are able to cope with a wider range of textures.[16]

Reliance on purees or smooth liquids for an extended period of time can create difficulty in moving on to textured or lumpy foods.[17] This can lead to sensitivity to, and refusal of, textured foods, and occasionally to intractable chewing difficulties, which may in turn trigger digestive problems. It can also result in chronic under- or overeating and prolonged dependence on bottle feeding, as well as impacting the sensory feedback that the child gets from food. This feedback tells us where food is in our mouth and how it is behaving. It allows us to distinguish between drinking applesauce and chewing a piece of cracker, and to apply different techniques to break them down and swallow them. This is a key part of a baby's learning to manage different textures safely. Commercial "baby foods" present additional drawbacks: They are generally less nutrient dense than table foods, so do not provide the same level of nutrition, and they tend to taste different from the same foods prepared at home.

Eating only soft food can affect the shaping of the structure of the oral cavity and the alignment of the teeth and may even influence the development of the airway.[18] Purees tend to be sucked into the mouth and then swallowed rapidly, without triggering, or requiring, chewing-related movements. In contrast, food in sticks or strips can be placed directly on the baby's gums, prompting up-down munching, as well as lateral tongue movements that are key to moving food around the mouth safely. The frequent gnawing, repetitive biting, and pulling movements that babies apply to strips of food promote jaw strength and grading, proprioceptive feedback, tongue mobility, and optimal chewing. These refined chewing skills help reduce the risk of choking and promote good digestion.

The baby's experience at mealtimes is relevant, too. Early exposure to textured foods makes eating more interesting, as does being allowed to decide what combinations of foods to try, rather than having a caregiver make that decision. This may explain why babies who follow BLW tend to enjoy meal-times more and eat a wider variety of foods[19] than babies who are fed purees, while also being less likely to become picky eaters.[20]

The case for self-feeding

With the change in the recommended minimum age for com-plementary feeding to 6 months, arguments for spoon feeding the majority of babies are hard to sustain.[21] Being spoon fed is a relatively passive experience for the infant. She is not required to exercise her core muscles or practice coordinating fine motor movements in order for food to arrive at her mouth. Generally, babies who are spoon fed are encouraged to look at their caregiver, rather than at the food, so there is little oppor-tunity for them to change the angle of their head or refocus their gaze. In contrast, the frequent hand-to-mouth practice that is key to self-feeding aids in improving aim, eye-hand coordination, visual skills, and motor strength, while simul-taneously engaging core muscles every time the baby leans forward to pick up food. Self-feeding also encourages midline orientation, through the use of both hands together in order to hold large pieces of food, or to turn foods over to examine them. This promotes an awareness of, and control over, the two sides of the body, which is essential for the development of symmetrical movements and to achieve balance. It also enables easy rotation of the core and the coordination of all four limbs. In short, while the focus of spoon feeding is on growth and nutrition, self-feeding expands the baby's expe-rience to encompass learning and development.

> I am impressed with how bringing food to midline
> influences posture and alignment.
>
> Lori Overland, speech-language pathologist

Feeding herself allows the baby to eat intuitively and manage her own appetite. This is especially important in babies with conditions such as Prader-Willi and Down syndrome, who are at particular risk for obesity and the multitude of further health issues that can result from overfeeding in infancy. It's all too easy for babies with feeding challenges to continue to be spoon fed for extended periods of time, primarily because of a lack of awareness among parents and professionals that self-feeding is a viable option. The longer babies are accustomed to being fed by an adult, the more difficult it becomes to encourage them to feed themselves, especially if they have low muscle tone, lack core strength, or are easily fatigued. It's not uncommon for some to be content to rely on an adult to feed them, or to continue to be fed by tube or bottle, way past the age when they could be eating independently—sometimes until 3 or even 5 years old—a situation that threatens their autonomy and growing independence.

Many babies have all their feeding decisions made for them because of a lack of belief that they can develop the necessary skills or make good choices for themselves. For those who, at 6 months, already have a feeding disorder, complicated medical history, issues with weight gain, or history of aversion to breast- or bottle feeding, the beginning of complementary feeding can be a real opportunity to provide an experience that is not only therapeutic but also positive and engaging. A baby-led approach has the potential to nullify learned negative responses and aversive feeding behaviors and give the baby back control over her eating, allowing her and her parents to enjoy mealtimes again.

> In my pediatric nutrition practice, I work with many children who have anxiety and fear around eating. Parents can see the difference that happens, often immediately, when their child is empowered to feed themselves. It makes me so happy to see a parent in awe of what their child is able to do when given the opportunity.
>
> Amy Manojlovski, registered dietitian

> All babies deserve the opportunity to feed themselves!
> Katie Ferraro, dietitian and baby-led weaning specialist

ADDIE'S STORY

Jill's account

ADDIE'S HISTORY

Addie is her parents' first child. She arrived early, at 24 weeks' gestation, weighing a little over 1 pound. She spent four months in a neonatal intensive care unit (NICU), during which she required mechanical ventilation and was diagnosed with chronic lung disease. She was discharged home still needing oxygen and on bottle feedings supplemented via a nasogastric tube. After two months at home she was fully bottle fed. Although she was unable to transition to breastfeeding, her mom provided Addie with her milk throughout Addie's first year. Addie also received medication for reflux; fortunately, a swallow study showed no signs of aspiration.

When Addie began oral feedings she found it difficult to accept the bottle and her parents had to rely on distraction in order to feed her. The family worked with a dietitian, to help address Addie's struggle with weight gain, as well as with a physical therapist and an occupational therapist. Her mom started to introduce solid foods when Addie was around 10 months old (which equated to 6 months' adjusted age, allowing for her prematurity) but she would turn her head and bat the spoon away, accepting only minimal amounts of commercial baby-food purees and cereal.

ADDIE'S FEEDING THERAPY INTERVENTION AND PROGRESS

I saw Addie for the first time when she was 1 year old (8 months adjusted). It was clear to me that she had developed a feeding aversion, almost certainly related to the necessary but frequent invasive oral procedures that were a feature of her prolonged NICU stay.

In our first session, having observed Addie's aversive responses when her mom tried to feed her, I wanted us to try offering her a pre-loaded spoon to hold for herself. The food needed to be something smooth and spreadable, so it would stay on the spoon easily. I asked what they had in the refrigerator and we opted for cream cheese and cake frosting. I think Addie's mom and babysitter thought I was a bit strange—but Addie didn't! She took to it right away, bringing the spoons pre-loaded with each food to her mouth by herself. She did the same with a silicone feeder filled with tangerine segments. We finished the session with her taking sips of orange juice from an open cup, which her mom helped her to hold.

Addie had a sensitive gag reflex and would later need to work on chewing skills, so for the first month we focused on smooth spreadable foods and table-food mashes. Her technique with pre-loaded spoons varied: She would sometimes put the handle in her mouth rather than the food side. She was also super-sensitive: sometimes even the smallest soft solid chunk would stimulate a gag, which then led to vomiting. This was challenging, given the concerns about her weight gain. She did like gnawing on a silicone feeder filled with orange slices, and was especially interested in drinking liquids, such as milk mixed with yogurt, from an open cup. We gradually increased the texture of her mashes, adding foods like guacamole, and then began introducing meltable solid foods, so she could work on taking bites and chewing. We slowly saw her start to demonstrate a munching pattern and begin to move her tongue sideways. In addition to the silicone feeder we offered her soft solid food pieces on a fork, placed at the level of her first molars, to encourage her to use her gums to chew. We attempted to use an oral motor kit, consisting of a vibratory base with a selection of textured attachments, to work on jaw strength and tongue movement, but Addie's sensitivity meant that she wasn't always accepting of it.

After the first month of ABLW, Addie was already beginning to use a pincer grasp to pick up and eat small pieces of banana. By her second month, she could manage foods like pumpkin bread, turkey lunch meat, a meatball, French-style green beans, cheese, orange segments, and steamed broccoli. After three months, her episodes of gagging and vomiting were much less frequent and she was able to progress to biting and pulling, with resistive strips of foods such as cheese. At first, she preferred to tear the strips into small pieces and then eat them, something that is quite usual when babies' biting skills are immature. To help her to learn, her mom or I would put our hand over Addie's, to help her to hold the strip steady in between her gums.

By the time she had been doing ABLW for around five months, Addie was able to take bites of large foods, such as whole bananas, although she was inclined to overstuff her mouth with smaller pieces. She went through a phase of throwing food but her parents created a "No, thank you" bowl and encouraged her to put into it any food she didn't want. Six months after beginning her ABLW journey, Addie had gone from refusing almost all food when it was offered to her on a spoon to complete self-feeding of table-food pieces, food strips, and bites of large foods.

For the next three months, we worked on improving Addie's jaw strength with resistive strips and refining her chewing skills using foods requiring more breakdown. During this time her mom and I liaised closely with the dietitian, adding ingredients such as nut butters, avocado, and full-fat milk products to her food, to help increase her calorie intake. She was drinking her mom's milk and whole cow's milk from a bottle, as well as a nutritional supplement drink, and she continued to enjoy assisted open-cup drinking of yogurt-type mixtures. Her pediatrician was pleased with her growth, which was steady if not rapid.

Addie was less successful with straw drinking and her progress with this skill was slower. We started with a therapeutic straw cup and worked on oral motor exercises to help with lip rounding and suction, for example, sucking applesauce out of a shortened straw. Eight months after beginning ABLW, she was successfully eating a variety of table foods of different shapes, sizes, and textures and had mastered straw drinking as well, so our focus moved to working on her speech and language development.

DISCUSSION

It is not uncommon for extremely pre-term infants to struggle with oral feedings, not least because many also have complicated medical histories. Feeding aversion occurs frequently. While Addie initially struggled to bottle feed and resisted adult-directed spoon feeding, the difference in her behavior when food was presented in a child-directed way was striking. After always having others control how and what she ate, this was the first time that she was in charge of feeding herself. Her rapid change over the course of six months was wonderful to witness. She went from a child who was fearful of eating to one who loved eating. The journey wasn't always smooth and she would have periods where she would gag and vomit at meals, throw food, and overstuff her mouth, but once her chewing skills became more refined she was able to enjoy a variety of table foods, and mealtimes became pleasant for the family. Much of Addie's success with ABLW can be attributed to her parents and babysitter, whose responsive approach and commitment to implementing the plan we devised resulted in a happy and safe eater.

ADDIE'S MOM'S PERSPECTIVE

Addie was born at 24 weeks' gestation weighing 1 pound 3 ounces. She had a long NICU stay that necessitated breathing and feeding tubes—and, unfortunately, all of the maintenance and discomfort that goes with them: insertion, removal, suctioning, and so on. As a result of her medical history, she developed issues with feeding, called an "oral aversion." Rather than enjoying a bottle or being spoon fed, she would turn her head, push food away, or occasionally gag and get sick. We used a nasogastric feeding tube for quite some time out of necessity, but Addie really turned the corner with her feeding issues when we began doing adapted baby-led weaning. During our first session with Jill, I almost instantly saw a shift in Addie's attitude toward food. Removing the spoon, which Addie had become defensive to, from the equation meant she now saw the food on her tray as an opportunity to play and explore, and inevitably ended up sampling it, too. Most important, ABLW gave her the power to determine what went in her mouth, on her own terms, which lessened her oral aversion and changed the dynamic at mealtime for the better.

5
.....

ABLW: Planning Ahead

The earlier preparation starts for the introduction of solid foods, the earlier a baby with additional needs is likely to become an independent eater. Understanding how foundational gross motor, fine motor, and oral motor skills develop in the first six months—and how they work together to support self-feeding with solid foods—will help ensure every newborn gets off to the best start. It will also help to prevent or minimize more difficult and complicated feeding problems farther down the line. A pre-feeding program and therapeutic feeding plan will form a key part of the lead-in to self-feeding with solid foods, but both of these rely on first building solid foundational skills right from birth. For parents, surrounding themselves with professionals who share their goals for their baby is an important first step.

Professional support

By the time they start solid foods, babies with neurological or motor challenges will likely already have a team of professionals supporting them. The job titles of the individuals, and their availability, will vary from country to country, but it's unlikely that any one professional will be able to provide for all the family's needs. Good communication and coordination among the members of the team and the baby's parents will help ensure that the guidance given is both appropriate and timely, and that decisions are made that support his nutrition, safety, skill development, autonomy, and enjoyment of mealtimes.

The exact makeup of the team will be determined by the baby's condition or diagnosis and will likely change over time, with the ebb and flow of his progress. Medical conditions that may impact feeding—whether developmental, functional, or structural—will require management and follow-up by one or more specialists. In addition to a general pediatrician and possibly a developmental pediatrician, the medical team may therefore include specialists in ear, nose, and throat disease (ENT); pediatric dentistry; gastrointestinal illnesses; neurological conditions; allergies; and disorders of the bones, muscles, lungs, heart, and other organs.

The baby is also likely to come under the care of a number of different therapists—for example, physical, occupational, developmental, and speech therapists; dietitian; and lactation consultant—whose role and level of input will vary according to his changing needs (see Appendix, page 245). Some babies will also require support from specialists in vision and hearing. In the USA, these services will usually be available, for 0- to 3-year-olds who have a disability or developmental delay, through a state Early Intervention program.[1] Wherever possible, two key members of the team should be a physical therapist and a feeding therapist, both of whom will need to be involved from the baby's birth. The feeding therapist is likely to be a speech pathologist but could equally be an occupational therapist. Ideally, they will have experience of both BLW and responsive feeding techniques, as well as the baby's specific diagnosis; if not, they should aim to work closely with members of the team who do.

It is helpful if the whole team is in agreement that exclusive breast- or formula feeding for the first six months is desirable and should be supported, and that the emphasis in the early weeks of complementary feeding should be on exploration, learning about foods, and honing feeding skills rather than on food intake. This allows everyone to focus on the baby's experience and opportunities for development. Parents (and some professionals) are often anxious about food volume and need reassurance that human milk and/or infant formula can meet all, or almost all, of a baby's nutritional needs for several months following the introduction of solid foods, freeing him up to learn about food and develop the skills he needs to become a safe eater. If there are concerns about weight gain or micronutrient intake (as in Addie's story, page 113), the involvement of a dietitian will help to ensure that the foods offered are nutrient rich, and that any necessary supplements are provided.

Building a solid foundation

A baby's ability to feed himself is underpinned by a range of foundational motor and oral skills (see chapter 3). Encouraging the development of these skills from birth will make an enormous difference to the progress the baby is able to make when he begins the transition to solid foods and may even help to avoid a delay in starting. There are three key areas parents can focus on during the first few months after birth to help ensure their baby is ready to start exploring solid foods as early as possible: mastery of early feeding skills, development of core strength, and sensory stimulation.

Supporting early feeding skills

Many of the eating skills that will be needed when solid foods are introduced have their roots in early milk feeding. Attention to enabling a baby who is at risk for feeding difficulties to feed as safely and effectively as possible at the breast or from a bottle therefore matters not just during the period of milk feeding but also later on.

Some babies who are born with medical, structural, or developmental conditions that affect feeding will initially need to be fed by tube, but even before they are ready to move on to oral feedings, they will ideally have input from a lactation consultant and/or a feeding therapist. These specialists will work together collaboratively, with the lactation consultant focusing on helping the mother establish and protect her milk supply, and the feeding therapist on assessing and promoting the baby's feeding skills. While the long-term goal is to discontinue tube feedings, maintaining them helps to ensure adequate nutrition and weight gain while the baby's ability to manage oral feedings is limited. This will tend to reduce the potential anxiety of caregivers and allow the baby to progress at his own pace.

Diane Bahr, a speech pathologist and feeding therapist, has created a detailed feeding checklist, extending from infancy to 24 months, to assist in identifying the presence or absence of necessary foundational feeding skills.[2] These include the baby's ability to locate the nipple with his mouth; to sustain a certain number of sucks in a sucking burst; and to coordinate sucking, swallowing, and breathing. Overland and Merkel-Walsh use a task analysis approach that takes this concept one step further, focusing on the specific skills needed for an oral sensory-motor task, such as breast- or bottle feeding, spoon feeding, chewing, or straw or cup drinking.[3] Those they identify for effective breast- or bottle feeding include mouth opening; tongue shape, position, and movement; and lip position. For the more complex skills of chewing, cup drinking, and taking food from a spoon, they highlight elements such as jaw stability, lip closure, and contraction of the cheek muscles. Breaking down a complex skill into its component parts like this can make it easier to pinpoint what an individual baby may be finding difficult. This allows for a more targeted approach to remedying the problem.

The identification of a baby's early feeding skills will usually be accompanied by an evaluation of oral structure and function and his ability to swallow (see page 100). Once the assessment is complete, safe ways to feed the baby will be

Pre-Feeding Skills

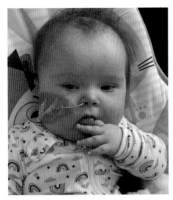

1 | Grace, 7 months, is finding out what her tongue can do, even though she is currently being fed via a tube.

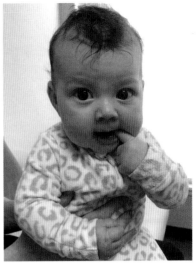

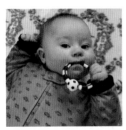

3 | Owen, 5 months, is practicing hand-to-mouth movements and munching while identifying the contours of his teething ring.

2 | Simone, 4 months, is using her fingers to create a mental map of the inside of her mouth and desensitize her gag reflex.

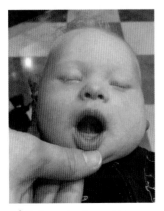

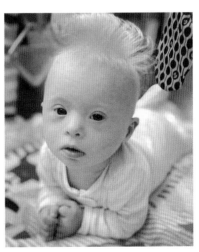

4 | At 4 weeks, the resting posture of Cassius's tongue is up in the roof of his mouth, helping to shape his palate.

5 | Cassius, 4 months, is practicing tummy time to work on strengthening the muscles of his neck, chest, and shoulders.

High Chair Essentials

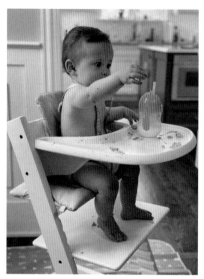

6 | Rewey, 13 months, is positioned ideally for safe self-feeding, with feet supported and hips, knees, and ankles at right angles.

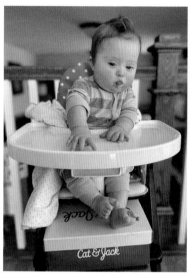

7 | The parents of Teddy, 7 months, have come up with a creative hack to support his feet until he grows a little.

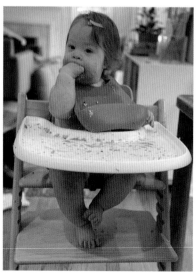

8 | Rose, 11 months, has a good sitting position, but this bib sometimes makes it difficult for her to see the food.

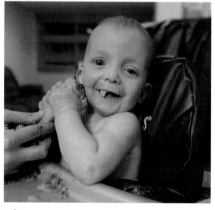

9 | Adiel, 8 months, has an insert in his high chair to provide the support he needs to sit stably.

Permission and Facilitation

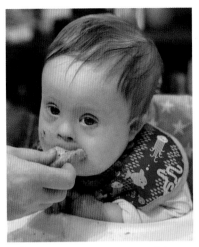

10 | Bodhi, 15 months (adjusted), is leaning forward toward this garlic bread, clearly demonstrating that he wants to try it.

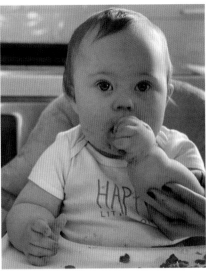

11 | Owen, 9 months, is bringing a food mash to his mouth, with some gentle facilitation from one of his parents.

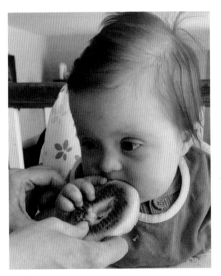

12 | Responsive facilitation: 8-month-old Teddy's parent is supporting his wrist and the bottom of a toasted bagel to help him bring it to his mouth.

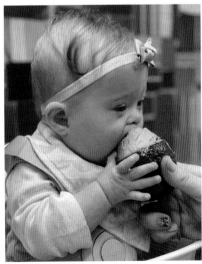

13 | Some parental help to manage the weight of this avocado means that Sophia, 8 months, can bring it to her mouth easily.

Teethers and Starter Strips

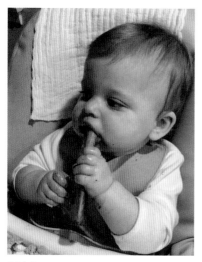

14 | Charlotte, 10 months, is honing her chewing and biting skills and hand-to-mouth movements on a smooth rib bone.

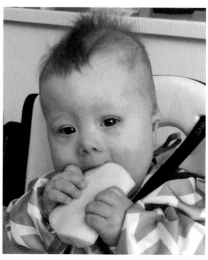

15 | Noah, 8 months, is using a mango pit to practice biting and chewing as well as using both of his hands together.

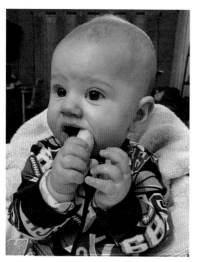

16 | Hayes, 6 months, has figured out how to position a thick strip of mango between his gums in order to chew it effectively.

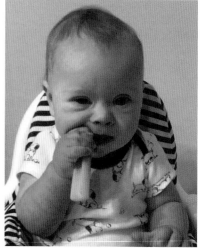

17 | Hudson, 7.5 months, is enjoying strengthening his jaw on this celery stick.

Spoons and Dippers

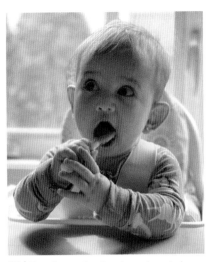

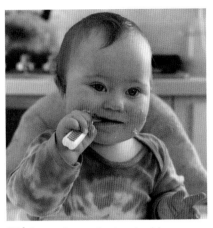

18 | Eva, 6 months, has been handed a pre-loaded spoon and is learning to use it to bring food to her mouth.

19 | Owen, 9 months, is using his spoon to work on his biting and chewing skills.

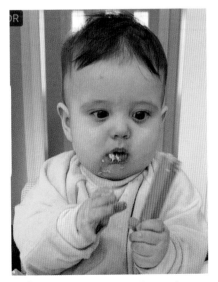

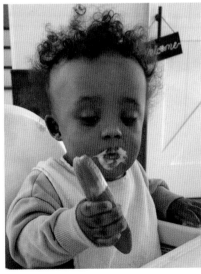

20 | At 7 months, Teddy is discovering that a carrot makes a great dipper for eating mashed sardines.

21 | Worth, 14 months, is studying his stick of cucumber to figure out why it tastes of yogurt.

Bridge Devices

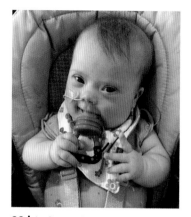

22 | At 6 months, Isla is using a feeder to learn to self-feed while the tube takes care of ensuring she has enough calories.

23 | When Noah, 5 months, munches on his silicone feeder, the food is forced out through the holes, so he can eat it.

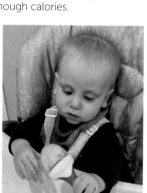

24 | Micah, 9 months, is about to bring a silicone feeder filled with rice cereal to his mouth for some chewing practice.

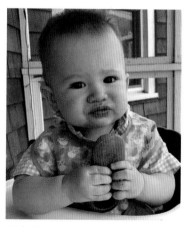

26 | Ethan, 17 months, is chewing on a straw filled with frozen puree, which gradually thaws, enabling him to eat it.

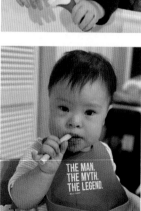

25 | Niko, 9 months, is working on hand-to-mouth skills while discovering just how cold a popsicle can be!

Large Foods

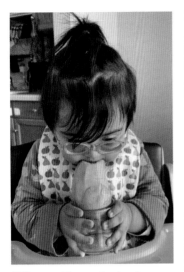

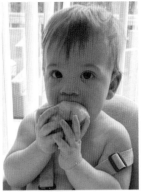

28 | Henry, 11 months, is eating a peach that has some of the skin left on, so gripping it is easier.

27 | Adira, 31 months, has her slippery mango supported in a drinking glass, which makes it easier to control.

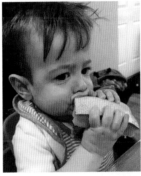

29 | This piece of melon is the perfect thickness for Luke, 10 months, to grasp while he discovers which side is edible.

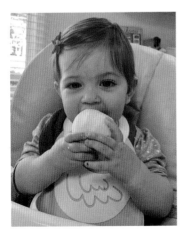

30 | Theodora, 9 months, is enjoying a whole apple with the core removed. This is safer than slices, which can snap easily.

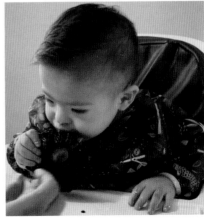

31 | Thiago, 17 months, is discovering the unique texture and taste of a portobello mushroom, enhancing his skills and his nutrition.

Looking and Learning

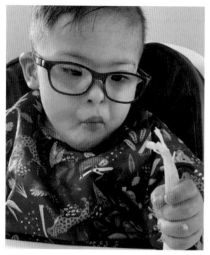

32 | Thiago, 17 months, is comparing the appearance of this stick of celery with the feel and taste of it in his mouth.

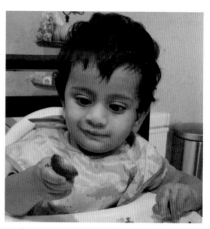

33 | Mustafa, 11 months, seems fascinated by the cut surface of his strawberry, which looks different from the outside.

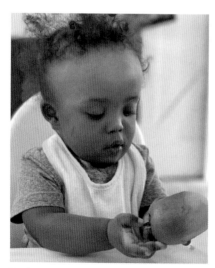

34 | Worth, 14 months, is coordinating his eyes and his hands to compare the peeled and unpeeled parts of this kiwi.

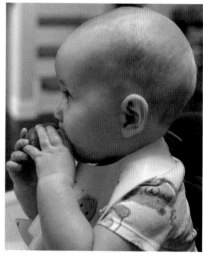

35 | Emmett, 6 months (adjusted), is watching his mom demonstrate how to eat a partially peeled kiwi.

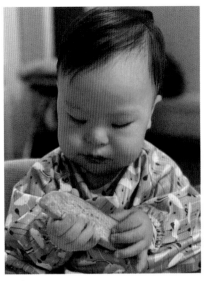

36 | Ethan, 12 months, is comparing the look and feel of the outer and inner surfaces of his baguette.

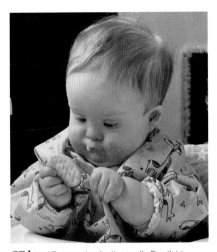

37 | At 13 months (adjusted), Bodhi is able to use his pointer finger to make sense of the dimpled surface of his cracker.

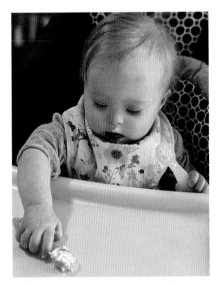

38 | Sophia, 12 months, must look downward and coordinate her head, eye, and hand movements to pick up her spoon.

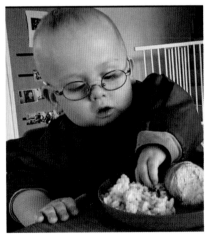

39 | Luan, 15 months, is focused on sampling some rice, steadying himself and reaching across midline to do it.

Bite Grading

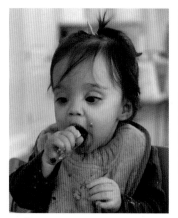

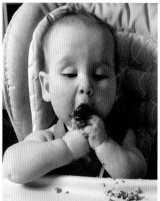

41 | This floret of broccoli is irregularly shaped, meaning that Ryan, 7 months, has to adjust his jaw opening to accommodate it.

40 | Viviana, 13 months (adjusted), is working on matching her mouth opening with the size of the bite.

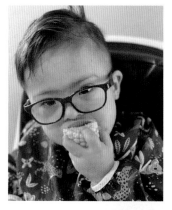

42 | Thiago, 17 months, is able to bite down easily on a corn cob when it's offered as a disk.

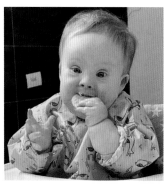

43 | At 13 months (adjusted), Bodhi has learned that he doesn't need to open his mouth very wide to bite a cracker.

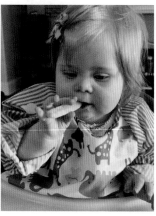

44 | Faith, 13 months, is using a very fine movement to hold this strip of banana without squishing it.

Picking Up and Taking

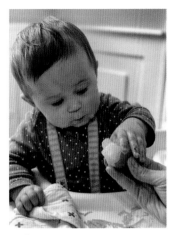

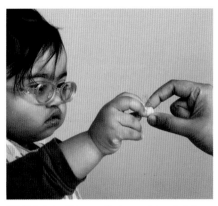

46 | To take this small piece of food, Adira, 31 months, is coordinating her eyes, her arm, and her fingers very precisely.

45 | Rewey, 11 months, is concentrating hard to take this kiwi from her parent's hand without dropping it.

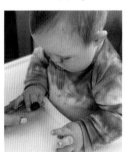

47 | Owen, 9 months, is looking down and attempting a pincer grasp to pick up a squashed blueberry from his parent's hand.

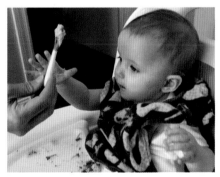

48 | Ava, 7 months, is reaching forward to grasp this pre-loaded spoon by the handle, so she can feed herself.

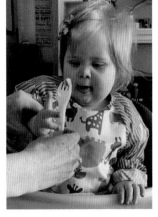

49 | At 13 months, Faith knows how to take food off a fork held by someone else and is learning how to grasp it herself.

Food Presentation

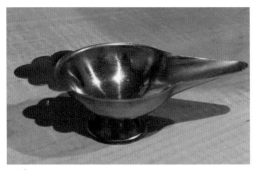

50 | Until the 18th century, papboats like this were in common use for feeding babies (see page 17).

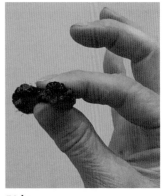

51 | The squish test: If a food can be squished like this, it is soft enough to be munched by a baby whose skills are still immature.

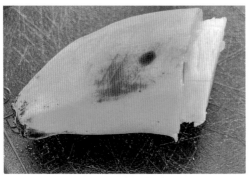

52 | A partially exposed banana helps babies learn to take graded bites.

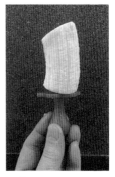

53 | Spearing a large piece of banana on a fork gives it a handle, so it can be held and gnawed easily.

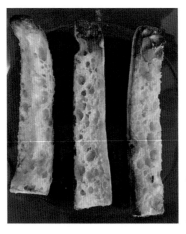

54 | Fingers of baguette, cut lengthways and toasted, offer a firmer texture than strips cut from a loaf of bread.

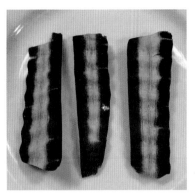

55 | A crinkle cutter can make slippery foods easier to hold, and some vegetables can yield fun surprises! These are purple carrots.

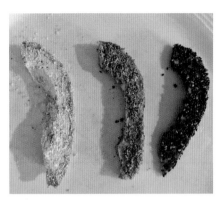

56 | These avocado strips have been rolled in (L to R) fine bread crumbs, ground flaxseed, and chia seeds to give them more grip.

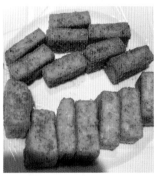

57 | Pan-fried tofu is a handy way to introduce protein and easy to cut into a shape that a baby can hold.

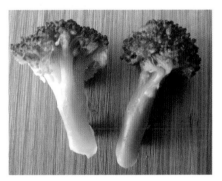

58 | Broccoli florets have their own built-in handle, especially when cut long.

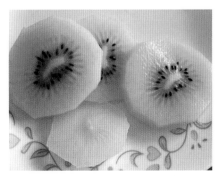

59 | Kiwis can be offered whole, as wedges, or sliced across into disks that are a great fit for little hands.

Drinking

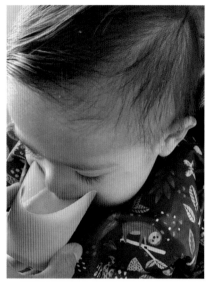

60 | A cut-out cup allows the parent of Thiago, 16 months, to better control the flow of liquid and see how much he is taking in.

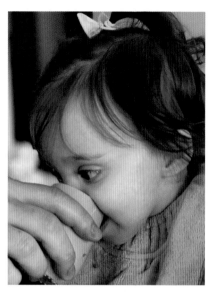

61 | At 13 months (adjusted), Viviana is adept at facilitated drinking from a regular open cup.

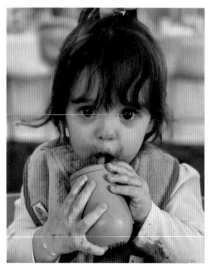

62 | At 13 months (adjusted), Viviana's twin sister, Liliana, is able to hold her straw cup and drink independently.

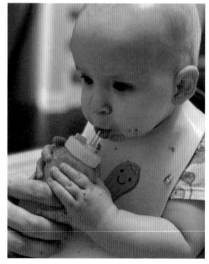

63 | Therapeutic straw drinking: See how Emmett, 6 months (adjusted), is using his cheek and lip muscles to create an effective vacuum.

Therapy

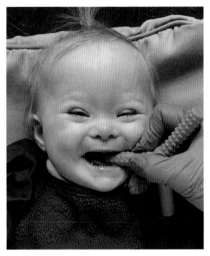

64 | The therapist is using a chewy tool to encourage Sophia, 11 months, to move her tongue sideways and chew effectively.

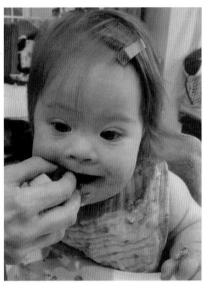

65 | A netted feeder containing a piece of chicken is helping Rose, 13 months, to make repeated chewing movements.

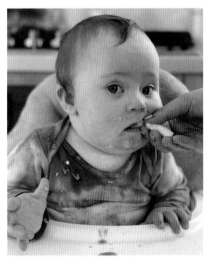

66 | The parent of Owen, 9 months, is using their fingers to help him learn how much to bite off at one time.

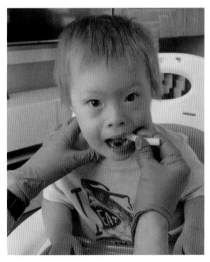

67 | The therapist is helping Evan, 30 months, to use his chewing surfaces to bite through a meltable snack food.

Skill Progression

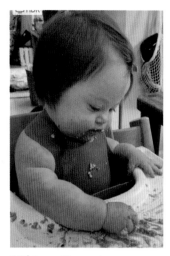

68 | Rose, 11 months, demonstrates her raking skills.

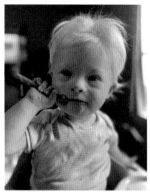

69 | By holding his green bean at the side of his mouth, Cassius, 10 months, learns to move his tongue to where the food is.

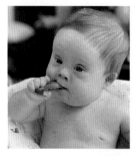

70 | Bodhi, 9 months (adjusted), shows off his resistive bite-and-pull skills on a strip of meat.

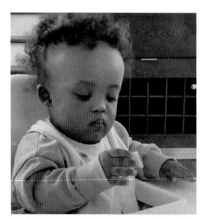

71 | Worth, 14 months, has picked up a piece of turkey, which he now has the complex chewing skills to manage.

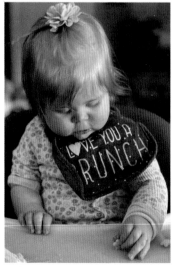

72 | At 13 months, Faith is able to pick up a tiny puff with a sophisticated pincer grip.

recommended, perhaps using devices such as a nipple shield or supplemental nursing system, or via experimentation with bottle nipples of varying flow, or thickening of feeds.

If specific feeding skills, such as grooving of the tongue or stability in the cheeks, are found to be absent, the feeding therapist will create an individualized program to work directly on these areas. This could be the type of pre-feeding program developed by Overland (see page 127) or another, similar approach. What matters is that it should be based on a solid understanding of the foundational feeding skills necessary at different points during the infant's feeding journey and on how to facilitate skills for the next step or level of difficulty.

Developing core strength

Strong core muscles are essential for postural stability and head control, which in turn are necessary for secure sitting, and for safe eating of solid foods. Babies who are carried in their parents' arms or in an upright sling for most of the day naturally exercise their core muscles in response to the parent moving around and changing position. However, in cultures where young babies spend a significant amount of time semi-reclining or on their back for play and sleep, those muscles are rarely engaged. One way to counter this is to ensure that they are spending equal amounts of time on their tummy (prone) as on their back during their waking hours. This is usually referred to as "tummy time," and it is especially important for babies whose overall muscle tone is low. Unfortunately, many babies don't like being placed on their tummy—most notably babies with reflux (see Rewey's story, page 82)—so it can be useful for parents to be shown ways to position and play with their baby in the prone position, as well as specific exercises and techniques,[4] all of which will help to engage and strengthen the necessary muscles.

In addition to helping to strengthen the muscles of the head and neck, tummy time also supports the development of a rounded head shape. When babies are positioned on their back or in a reclining seat, especially one with movement, such as a swing, their head tends to remain in the position that is most comfortable for them. This causes uneven pressure on the skull, which can lead to flattening of the side or back of the head—a condition known as plagiocephaly (an added complication for Rewey, see page 82). It can also affect the shape of the face and the oral cavity,[5] potentially contributing to chewing, swallowing, and breathing difficulties. Frequent bouts of tummy time help to prevent the bones of the skull from becoming misshapen in this way.

Stimulating the senses

Well before they're ready to eat or drink anything other than milk, babies are building a store of sensory experiences that they will draw on when they encounter solid food. Right from birth, they can start to experience the feel of a wide variety of materials on their hands, arms, and body—not just soft-touch and plastic toys but another person's skin, wood, silky fabrics, moving air, grass, feathers, and so on. They can also begin to distinguish properties such as wet and dry or warm and cold and to identify different shapes. As they develop more refined hand-to-mouth movements, they can move on to exploring safe objects with their mouth as well as their hands, discovering oral sensations of shape, texture, and temperature—and, of course, taste.

The touch receptors in the mouth develop very early in fetal life, enabling the newborn to search for and latch on to his mother's breast. At birth he will already be used to licking and sucking his hands in a generalized way and will gradually move to more discriminative mouthing, with his fingers inside of his mouth, by around 4 to 6 months old. If he is offered chewy toys, he will discover how to use them to reach farther back inside his mouth, triggering important feeding reflexes (see page 52) and assisting with mouth mapping (see page 64).

Repetition of grasping, mouthing, and hand-to-mouth movements is a great foundation for self-feeding, not only because it allows the baby to practice basic feeding actions but because it helps him to create links between how things feel on the skin of his fingers and palm and how they feel inside his mouth. This allows him to anticipate how an object, or a food, will behave when he tries to bite or chew it, which is hugely important for safe eating. These experiences also stimulate his curiosity, which is a key element of a positive transition to solid foods. Avoiding hands-in swaddling and mittens (especially when the baby is awake) and instead allowing babies to have their arms and hands free for hand-to-mouth exploration of toys and other objects is important for many aspects of their development, including feeding.

A pre-feeding program: what and why

A pre-feeding program is a tailored therapeutic exercise plan to support feeding, based on a task analysis (see page 122) of the underlying movements of the lips, cheeks, jaw, and tongue. It uses a variety of techniques, including oral exercises and transition devices and is designed to facilitate oral sensory awareness and skill development and to promote the foundational skills necessary for safe eating *in advance* of those skills being put into practice with food. Babies who show sensory-based feeding aversion in the first six months, perhaps because of reflux or as a result of a choking or other incident (see page 95), but who do not have structural or developmental issues, may not require a pre-feeding program, since their neurological and feeding skill development will usually be in line with that of their typically developing peers. However, those who are subject to long-term tube feeding may benefit from such a program, to increase and maintain their tolerance of oral sensations and to work on the foundational oral skills necessary to support chewing.

A pre-feeding program should begin before solid foods are introduced (as with Sophia; see page 133) but will likely continue alongside a therapeutic feeding plan (see page 129). In either case, the pre-feeding exercises will always be focused on developing more advanced skills than the baby is currently using to eat, thereby preparing him ahead of time for tackling more complex foods. Tools used as part of a pre-feeding program will be specifically tailored to the needs of the individual baby. They may include, for example, a specialized tongue depressor tip to work on bilabial closure (the bringing together of the lips to help produce sounds like *muh*, *buh*, and *puh*), differently shaped silicone chews and teethers (as demonstrated by Sophia in photo 64) to help develop jaw strength and tongue mobility, and soft-tipped wand-shaped tools to encourage cheek resistance. (See Resources, page 259, for further information.) Overland's sensory-motor approach[6] is comprehensive, systematic, and infant-oriented, and it pairs particularly well with adapted BLW. Using this approach, the therapist will create a tailored program based on the individual baby's needs. Crucially, they will show the baby's parent how to carry out the exercises so they can be practiced at home. This is essential if the program is to be effective. Here are some examples of Overland's pre-feeding exercises:

- For an infant who is having breast- or bottle feeding difficulties and is still being tube fed, Overland might suggest an exercise known as tongue grooving, in which the therapist or parent places a gloved finger at the tip of the baby's tongue and applies firm downward pressure along the midline to a point halfway back, in an effort to create a concave shape. This promotes the tongue position necessary to transport milk to the back of the mouth for swallowing. Tongue grooving can be helpful when milk is spilling from a baby's mouth during feeding, associated with either a neurological issue or a structural anomaly, such as a tongue-tie.

- As a baby approaches the beginning of solid food introduction, Overland might recommend the use of two soft-tipped therapeutic tools or two gloved fingers placed against the sides of the baby's tongue and then firmly stroked forward from the back of the tongue on both sides simultaneously, to draw out the tip. This encourages elongation of the tongue, which is a prerequisite for the side-to-side movements necessary for chewing (see "Learning to chew," page 58).

- For a baby who has started solid foods and can break down a soft food strip or lumpy foods with a munching action but cannot yet chew more complicated foods (such as chicken), pre-feeding exercises aimed at promoting a diagonal chewing movement and pointing of the tip of the tongue may be appropriate. For example, this might consist of placing a silicone chew on the baby's outermost lower incisor (or the place where that tooth will appear) and rolling it to the area of the first molar on the same side. This will encourage sideways movements of the tongue in preparation for foods that require more refined chewing.

An additional and integral part of Overland's pre-feeding program is the chewing hierarchy. This consists of four steps that gradually facilitate effective and more complex jaw and tongue movements, to enable safe eating of both simple and more texturally complex foods.[7] Achieving this chewing transition, from munching through to an adult rotary chewing pattern, will usually involve a combination of pre-feeding and therapeutic feeding activities. The goal is for the baby to be able to achieve dissociation of the lips, tongue, and jaw, so that he can use his tongue by itself to move food to his gums for chewing, use his lips independently of his tongue to remove food from a spoon and drink from a straw, and make appropriately graded jaw movements to bite a piece off a large item of food.

Devising a therapeutic feeding plan

Using food in a tailored way to help a baby develop his feeding skills has been termed "therapeutic feeding."[8] A therapeutic feeding plan begins at birth, or as soon as anticipated or actual feeding difficulties are identified. Its purpose is to help babies acquire the skills they need to ensure safe eating and adequate nutrition, as well as culturally appropriate mealtime behavior. The plan will initially focus on safe liquid intake, via breast- and/or bottle feeding, and then begin working on developing skills for the safe management of solid foods. It may be implemented on its own or in conjunction with a pre-feeding program (see page 126). Therapeutic feeding techniques used in early infancy may consist of simple changes to the baby's or mother's position to assist breast- or bottle feeding, but, as solid foods are introduced, they will address chewing skills, with food cut into specific shapes, like strips and cubes, along with strategic placement of those foods on the gums.

Part of the focus of the feeding plan will be to prevent or correct compensatory eating patterns. These are strategies commonly adopted by babies who find certain actions difficult, which allow them to use familiar movements instead. For example, babies may use their tongue to mash food against their palate rather than moving it to their gums, or they may bring their tongue forward in an immature suckling movement when drinking from a straw instead of using their lips and cheek muscles. A feeding therapist can identify these atypical strategies and suggest ways to avoid or overcome them, as well as help parents select foods of textures, shapes, and sizes that are appropriate and safe for the baby's developing skills.

An approach to the introduction of solid foods that is based on sensory-motor activities and a chewing hierarchy is an excellent fit with adapted baby-led weaning. The combination of task analysis, a pre-feeding program, and a therapeutic feeding plan with adapted BLW will enable the baby to feed himself with food shapes and textures that are appropriate to his skill level, while simultaneously ensuring that necessary and foundational oral motor skills are present. This creates an ideal pathway to independent eating. While such an approach has advantages for babies facing a variety of feeding challenges, neurodiverse babies, in particular, will benefit from this sort of comprehensive plan, which allows them to explore and eat solid foods at their own pace.

Determining readiness for solid foods

Babies whose feeding development is atypical, owing to structural, tonal, and/or neurological anomalies, may not be ready to start eating solid foods at 6 months. However, recognizing the point at which an individual baby is ready to begin the transition is important: too early and eating may not be safe; too late and crucial learning time will be lost.

Most often, the biggest delaying factor to beginning solid feeding using an adapted baby-led weaning approach is lack of the motor skills necessary for the baby to be able to keep his head and trunk upright in a supported sitting position, so that he can bring food items to his mouth accurately and safely.

The significance of the tongue-thrust reflex

It is often thought that the persistent presence of the tongue-thrust reflex (see page 70) is a sign that it's too early to start solid foods. This notion likely stems from the days of parent-directed spoon feeding of babies who, we now know, were too young to be given those foods. When complementary feeding was common from 3 or 4 months of age (or even younger), parents were advised to expect their baby to use his tongue, initially, to eject the food; they were told that, if they persevered, he would "get used to the spoon." In fact, this supposed learning was simply the extrusion reflex spontaneously disappearing. From the 1980s onward, when the recommended starting age changed to 4 to 6 months, the natural integration of the reflex during this period was considered one of several markers of a baby's readiness for solid foods.

For the majority of babies, the tongue-thrust reflex is no longer evident at 6 months; however, it often lingers in babies whose development is atypical, which can make attempts at spoon feeding futile. But the persistence of the reflex need not be an obstacle to the introduction of solid foods using a baby-led approach. With ABLW, food exploration and skill learning are the focus, not intake. Increasing numbers of therapists share the view that babies for whom this reflex is still involuntary can nevertheless be encouraged to explore food strips and large foods in order to develop their dexterity and familiarity with food and promote chewing skills.

This is where the combined efforts of the physical therapist and the feeding therapist will be key, so that work on developing core strength can take place, in parallel with a pre-feeding program, to ensure that solid foods can be introduced in a timely manner. For babies whose core strength is good but who lack the hand-to-mouth skills to self-feed independently, this interim period is the time when ABLW's transitional phase with food exploration comes into its own.

The need for flexibility over the timing of the first solid foods can be confusing for parents, when they know that 6 months is the recommended age for their introduction. They may be concerned that their baby will lack important micronutrients or miss opportunities for experiencing potential allergens. Their unease can be made worse if the baby's medical team recommends starting at the six-month mark (or earlier), without recognizing that the baby lacks the necessary skills to support a safe transition. Communication between the medical and developmental teams, dietitians, and the baby's parents or other caregivers is therefore crucial.

The keys to supporting a baby with feeding challenges to transition to solid foods are patience and positivity. Progress may sometimes seem agonizingly slow, with the baby staying in one phase for an extended period. For example, he may spend a long time eating mashed soft solid foods off a pre-loaded spoon before being able to pick up those same foods, as mashes or pieces, from his high chair tray. Babies themselves rarely give up, but they need the positive support of those around them if they are to make the best progress.

SOPHIA'S STORY

Jill's account

SOPHIA'S HISTORY

Sophia is her parents' third child. She was diagnosed with Down syndrome at birth. She was also found to have two small heart defects (patent ductus arteriosus and patent foramen ovale), both of which resolved spontaneously by the time she was 3 months old. She required formula supplementation for a few days after birth because of a Rhesus blood incompatibility but was receiving only her mom's milk from day five.

I met Sophia and her mom when Sophia was 5 weeks old. At that time she preferred to have her mom's milk from a bottle and would feed only briefly at the breast, tiring easily. We used a nipple shield to help her latch and would drip milk onto it to entice her. Her mom worked hard to stimulate and maintain her milk supply, and, when Sophia started to nurse for longer periods of time at the breast, she rented a digital scale so that she could monitor milk transfer. By 3 months, Sophia was having all her feeds at the breast.

SOPHIA'S FEEDING THERAPY INTERVENTION AND PROGRESS

During Sophia's first six months, I gave her parents a pre-feeding program of exercises to do with Sophia that would help work on jaw strength, tongue movement, and a closed-mouth resting posture (to promote optimal shaping of the palate). I also explained the importance of Sophia's spending time on her tummy every day. These measures would ensure that she developed a strong foundation, so that she could start solid foods right on time.

Sophia began adapted BLW at 6 months, when she was still physically quite tiny. Her first challenge was how to see over the top of her high chair tray! Her mom had to place a box under Sophia's bottom so she could reach the food easily. We began with starter food strips of carrot, pepper, and cucumber, and Sophia took to it right away. She needed support only a few times to get the food to her mouth and then she began doing it by herself, spontaneously gnawing on the strip. We also offered her a thickened liquid from an open cup, which she managed with a little help. Next, we introduced her to gnawing on a pineapple core and eating blackberries in a silicone feeder, both of which she managed with two hands. We also began offering her spoons pre-loaded with textured soft solid mashes, such as guacamole.

Sophia's therapy is ongoing. At 8 months, she is self-feeding with table-food mashes from the silicone feeder and can pick up a pre-loaded spoon from her tray and get it to her mouth. She is happy to have small pieces of steamed pear placed on the lateral surface of her gums with a fork (therapeutic fork feeding; see page 204) and is able to munch them effectively. She has been working on chewing with frozen straws and is starting to take bites of soft solid strips of foods, such as avocado. However, she is not yet able to separate (dissociate) the movements of her tongue from those of her jaws and lips, so she turns toward where the strip is placed. She can gnaw on a whole avocado with the peel removed from the top, drink independently from a straw cup, and use an open cup with help. She continues to breastfeed, with one bottle of expressed milk each day. Her mom has already introduced her to all nine major allergens, and her ABLW journey is off to a great start!

DISCUSSION

Two months into ABLW and Sophia is rocking it! I attribute her rapid progress to a few factors: First, the work started when she was a newborn. That gave us plenty of time to prepare for solid foods through establishing breastfeeding, introducing frequent periods of tummy time, creating a pre-feeding program—which we implemented from 5 weeks—and assembling a developmental team. The team consisted of a physical therapist, an occupational therapist, a developmental therapist, a dietitian, and me as the feeding therapist. Second, an early start with physical therapy helped Sophia establish a strong foundational gross motor base, which meant that she was able to begin solids right at 6 months. Third, Sophia's parents were relaxed about introducing solid foods, having navigated it successfully with their first two children. They were also fully committed to implementing all the techniques and strategies that I and the other members of the team suggested.

At the time of writing, we are still working on Sophia's oral motor skills, refining her chewing with strips and food placement and improving her jaw stability with open-cup drinking. At 8 months she truly loves food and enjoys sharing meals with her family. Her transition to solids has been stress-free and her self-feeding skills are closely in line with her neurotypical peers.

Sophia's mom's perspective

I met with Jill after Sophia was born and diagnosed with Down syndrome. Until then, I had no idea what adapted baby-led weaning was. Sophia and I struggled with nursing and needed help, so it was a bonus that Jill was a lactation consultant as well as a speech pathologist. After three months I was successfully breastfeeding Sophia, so we began the discussion about solids and what we would do. I was surprised and wasn't sure what to think, initially, when Jill explained that my baby would be able to feed herself when she started solids.

At 6 months Sophia was showing signs of being ready and had the stability to begin. Jill explained how we would start and advance to the next stages. Day One of ABLW, Sophia was offered carrot sticks sized to fit in her hand, along with applesauce thinned with my milk in a cup. On that first day, she quickly picked up on the idea that when I put a food stick in her hand, she was to bring it to her mouth and chew on it. Her figuring it out so quickly, and on her own, was the biggest moment. My older two children hadn't done this at 6 months old, and they didn't have Sophia's challenges.

In the two months since we have started solids, Sophia has eaten about twenty different foods, including all of the allergens and most of the common fruits, vegetables, and meats. We are working on the next step of her being able to pick food off her plate instead of it being placed in her hand. Adapted baby-led weaning provides Sophia the jumpstart of fine motor skills along with the jaw strengthening she will need to help her develop other skills and be an active participant in her feedings.

6
.....

Getting Set Up

The setting for mealtimes is as important to a baby's learning as the meal itself. She needs to be comfortable, able to reach the food easily, and free to concentrate on what she's doing. She also needs company while she eats—and her caregivers need to be ready for some mess! This chapter looks at some of the practicalities of implementing an adapted form of baby-led weaning with a baby who is likely to need extra support to enable her to become an independent eater.

Seating matters

Selecting the right seating for babies who are going to be feeding themselves is extremely important, especially for those with motor and posture issues. Babies who have low muscle tone or neurological conditions need to be securely positioned in order to eat effectively and safely. Some babies, such as those with Down syndrome, tend to be smaller than their peers, which adds to the challenge of choosing a suitable seat. Early input from a physical therapist may help to ensure self-feeding gets off to a good start.

The primary consideration when deciding on seating is postural stability. While a baby doesn't need to be able to sit independently on the floor in order to be ready for solid foods, if she is not stable in a supported sitting position, doesn't have adequate head control, and struggles to bring her hand to her mouth without falling to the side, she should be allowed time to improve her core strength before embarking on this new adventure—even if this means delaying the start. Molded seats can seem to provide a solution to the problem of stability, but they are not ideal for babies, especially while eating. Because of the way they are shaped, these chairs cause the baby's pelvis to tilt back, making it hard for her to achieve a fully upright posture. The result is a rounded trunk and unnatural positioning of the head and neck. Maintaining this position is tiring for the baby and makes reaching for food difficult. It also prevents effective jaw and tongue movements and may affect digestion. All of this is especially unhelpful for babies who have low muscle tone or other physical challenges.[1]

In most situations, the best place for the baby to sit for self-feeding will be in a high chair. However, some babies may initially feel unsafe in a situation where they aren't in bodily contact with a parent. This may be simply because the situation is new, or it may be connected with one or more unpleasant or painful experiences associated with eating or with having been away from mom or dad. In these cases, it may be best to start with the baby on her parent's lap when at the table and slowly make the transition to the high chair as she becomes more familiar with what is going to happen. This may also be helpful as a temporary measure for babies who are very small, for whom conventional high chairs are not a good fit.

A good high chair is an excellent investment, especially if it is designed to accommodate the child as she grows.[2] While these chairs tend to be costly, they are usually worth the expense, as optimal seating can hugely influence the ability to self-feed. A chair with a tray is generally the best option for a baby's early forays into the world of solid foods. However, it's worth bearing in mind that the eventual goal is for her to share the same eating surface as the rest of the family. This will give her a better view of what, and how, everyone else is eating, which will motivate her to be adventurous with new foods. It will also enable her to feel part of what's going on and to join in the general conversation. A detachable tray will allow her to continue using the same seat when she graduates to eating at the big table, while also making it easier to lift her in and out and to clean up after meals.

Postural stability can be either enhanced or undermined by the design and construction of the high chair. The first consideration is support for the baby's feet, as this gives stability to the whole body. (Think of sitting on a bar stool with your feet dangling, then reaching for your drink!) An adjustable footrest that, when positioned correctly, allows for the baby's feet to be planted flat, with 90-degree angles at the hip, knee, and ankle, is ideal. While there are hacks for a footrest that can be created with, for example, a box and some tape (as with Teddy, photo 7), babies with neurodevelopmental challenges will benefit from the firm support of a plastic or wooden footrest (see Rewey, photo 6), which will provide better feedback through their feet and legs, helping them to balance and promoting physiologically correct positioning of the pelvis.

The height of the tray (or table) in relation to the seat of the high chair is another feature crucial to eating stability and comfort. The baby needs to be able to reach the eating surface without having to alter the position of her trunk or her head. It's common to see babies having to lift their whole arm—and even their shoulder, meaning they have to tilt themselves sideways—in order to reach their food. This seriously challenges the baby's balance and is awkward and tiring. (If you've ever been the one who had to sit on the low stool to eat at a family gathering because there were no more chairs you'll know what that's like.) The problem is made worse if the chair has high sides that prevent the baby from moving her arms easily. Ideally, the top of the rim of the high chair tray, or the surface of the table, should be at a level somewhere between the baby's belly button and her nipples, so that she can reach effortlessly for whatever is placed in front of her. If the tray or table cannot be lowered sufficiently, the answer may be to put something firm and flat under the baby's bottom, to raise her body to the required height. In that case, don't forget to also raise the footrest!

If the seat of the high chair is too wide or slippery, the baby may struggle to stay upright. In many cases, a rolled-up towel around her hips or some anti-slip gripper matting under her bottom will be enough to provide the necessary support. Other babies (such as Adiel, see page 149 and photo 9) may need a specially designed insert.[3] In general, a plain wooden or solid plastic chair will be the simplest to adapt—with the added advantage of being easier to clean than a padded one.

Preparing for the mess

When babies first begin to explore food they inevitably create some mess. There's a good chance that, during the course of a meal, some food will make its way onto all nearby surfaces, including the baby herself (arms, face, clothes, hair), the high chair, and the floor. All this can happen long before she chooses to take any of it to her mouth, and it's an important part of her learning. Freedom to make some mess also helps to reduce the likelihood that a baby will develop an aversion to the tactile sensations involved in handling food.

At first, dropping food is accidental, but even when it starts to be done on purpose it's not intended to be annoying. Sometimes it's a way of avoiding eating, but mostly it's just a feature of the discoveries the baby is making and her changing skill level. While it can be frustrating for parents or caregivers, pressure-free, messy food experiences are hugely important for a baby's development because they activate all her senses and stimulate her to try new ways to problem solve. The best approach is to expect some mess and plan ways to make the cleanup as easy as possible rather than try to restrict the baby's activities.

Coping with mealtime mess: tips for parents

Here are some tips for keeping cleanup quick and easy while allowing your baby freedom to explore and experiment:

- Keep a pair of footie pajamas just for mealtimes, or, if the room is warm enough, undress your baby down to just a diaper for eating.

- Plan bath time and dressing for the day or night for after breakfast or dinner, not before.

- Try a variety of bibs to find one that works for you and your baby.

- Put a clean "splat mat" under your baby's chair, so thrown food can be picked up and placed back on the tray during the meal and then gathered up easily at the end.

- Model putting unwanted food on a plate and encourage your baby to do the same.

- Try to avoid wiping your baby's face or hands during the meal. This will be irritating for her (imagine how you would feel if someone did it to you!) and may make her reluctant to touch the food. Just have one big cleanup at the end.

There is a variety of gadgets on the market that promise to contain dropped food, which you may find helpful—if not at home, then perhaps when eating out. They may also be useful in daycare and clinic settings or at the house of a friend or relative who can't tolerate a mess. If you are in a situation where you absolutely have to avoid food being spread around and are unable to delay the mealtime (or offer a milk feed instead), there are a few things you can do to keep the chaos to a minimum. For example, you might choose firmer, drier, or less slippery foods or prepare thicker mashes that won't easily come off a pre-loaded spoon. You could opt for a pre-loaded fork or large food, like a partially peeled pear, and encourage your baby to lean forward to eat it while you hold it. A silicone feeder or pouch may occasionally provide a compromise, allowing her to feed herself even though she can't see the food properly. If you have to spoon feed her for this one meal, so be it (although that, too, can be messy)—just take care to follow her cues.

It can be useful for parents to discuss with their feeding therapist the best clothing for their baby to wear at mealtimes. While washability is a given, there are some other considerations that may not be obvious. For example, long sleeves risk not only getting covered in food but also catching on stray pieces of food, resulting in more of it ending up on the floor. A bib may seem like the obvious answer but, depending on the design and the fabric, some bibs can seriously restrict a baby's movements, leading to frustration. Smock-type coveralls often swamp smaller babies, with long sleeves adding unnecessary bulk or covering the baby's hands. Bibs with a pelican-style pocket for catching food can be useful, but those made of rigid material will tend to make movement difficult. In particular, as demonstrated by Rose (photo 8), the pocket can get stuck between the baby and the tray, restricting the baby's view of the food and her ability to reach it. Many parents decide that bare arms are the best option, with a simple bib that goes over the baby's head like a shirt or fastens with Velcro behind the neck and fits flush against her chest.

Shared mealtimes

One of the most important aspects of helping babies learn to eat is making mealtimes a shared experience. Whenever possible, babies and their parents (or other caregivers) should aim to eat together rather than the parent watching the baby eat (or vice versa). Eating together makes mealtimes into a social event, in which communication skills and language are fostered and eating skills modeled; it can also help to retain the baby's interest in the meal for longer.

Shared mealtimes mean that the baby is exposed to a variety of foods presented in the way that is usual in that family. In fact, long before a baby starts solid foods, exposure to the sights, sounds, and smells of the kitchen and the table will stimulate her awareness and understanding of food. She'll learn what's safe to eat, and she'll make connections among appearance, smell, taste, and texture, so that she comes to recognize familiar foods and know what to expect from them.

Sitting with others at the table and watching what they do shows the baby how to tackle foods of varying sizes and shapes and prompts her to want to try it herself. She's less likely to be confused or worried by a new texture or shape if she's exposed to a wide variety from the outset, through sharing with others. For example, she can be given the opportunity to take a bite from a whole banana or a banana spear, pick up small pieces of banana, or manage mashed banana offered on a pre-loaded spoon or placed on her tray. She'll also be more eager to taste something unfamiliar if she sees others eating it first. There is nothing more powerful and effective in motivating a baby to try a new food than watching the people who matter to her eating and enjoying it.

> After the first few months Evan was able to self-feed with most of the same foods that our family ate for meals and that his peers had at daycare. It's been a great experience and he's continuing to refine his skills every day!
>
> Carolyn, mother of Evan, who has Down syndrome

Scheduling mealtimes at home

In the beginning, it's not necessary for your baby to be hungry in order for her to join you at mealtimes. It's her exposure to food and to others eating that matters; her nutrition will continue to be provided by her milk feeds. But she does need to be awake and alert rather than sleepy, so that she can enjoy, and take full advantage of, this new experience. For the same reason, you wouldn't offer her a new toy when she was tired and needing a nap. With this in mind, in the run-up to starting solid foods you may want to review how your mealtimes currently fit with her feeding and sleeping pattern. If, like lots of parents, you tend to eat while your baby is napping, that will need to change if she's to be interested and motivated when she joins you at the table. It may be that her routine can be tweaked, but it's equally likely that you'll need to amend your schedule. If you can't share every mealtime with her, try to make a point of eating something alongside her whenever she's eating, even if it's just a few bites.

Minimizing distractions

As far as possible, the environment at mealtimes should be low-key and calm—especially for a baby who is hypersensitive to external stimuli or easily distracted. Televisions, smart speakers, and cell phones need to be switched off and toys and pets removed from the immediate area. Keeping interruptions to a minimum helps, too—for example, by placing all the food on the table before the meal begins so that everyone can stay seated.

A plain eating surface will help the baby to focus on eating; patterned tray covers and tablecloths may seem attractive, but they tend to take the baby's interest away from the food, as well as making it difficult for her to distinguish it clearly. A dark surface can provide a better contrast to some foods than a white one; some high chair manufacturers make trays and tray covers in a selection of colors as well as white.

Bowls can be a help or a hindrance. For babies with gross and fine motor challenges, being able to push the food against the side of a suction-based bowl or plate can make picking up individual pieces easier. However, for many babies, especially at first, bowls and plates will be a distraction and will likely end up on the floor. In this instance, it's preferable to offer the food directly, for the baby to pick up from the caregiver's hand or to place it on the tray in front of her.

While company at mealtimes is a good thing, babies don't need cheerleaders! Too much enthusiasm or praise can be overwhelming or lead to distorted associations between emotions and food (see page 34), while coaxing tends to dampen their natural curiosity. Quiet encouragement, support, space, and time are all that's needed.

How often and for how long?

Parents are often given advice about starting solids that we now know is unnecessary. For example, they're frequently advised to limit the number of meals they offer to their baby, beginning with one meal a day and working up to three by the time the baby is a year old. They are also commonly still told to leave a gap of several days after offering a new food before introducing another. Except in the case of a baby who is under the care of a pediatrician and/or dietitian for a digestive disorder or possible allergy, neither of these precautions is necessary when solid foods are introduced at around 6 months (adjusted as appropriate for prematurity). By this age the baby's digestive system is robust and ready to digest a range of foods—and, if she feeds herself, she is very unlikely to eat more than she needs. There is no need to worry, either, about whether she will eat enough. She can continue getting the nutrition she needs from human milk and/or infant formula (with supplements if needed) for at least the next few months; her solid meals are about exposure and exploration, not volume.

It can help to think of the baby's milk feedings as her source of food and the shared mealtimes as an opportunity for play, socializing, learning, and skill development. There's no more reason to restrict mealtimes than to restrict her opportunity to play with toys. Indeed, the more practice she has at exploring different types of food with her hands and mouth the quicker she will gain the skills she needs to become an efficient self-feeder. This is especially true for babies with motor challenges, who will benefit enormously from frequent use of their core muscles and practice at hand-to-mouth movements.

A mealtime should continue for as long as the baby is interested and happy—regardless of how much she has or hasn't eaten. Initial food explorations may last as little as 5 minutes before she announces that she's done. She may indicate that she has finished by turning away from presented food, banging her hands on her tray, or sweeping or dropping food onto the floor. If these subtle cues are missed, she may start fussing verbally or even crying, which is a signal to end the meal immediately. With repeated exposure and practice, she will soon be happy to spend anywhere from 10 to 30 minutes, and possibly longer, at the table. At the same time, she will discover that eating is a fun activity and that it fills her belly. Mealtimes will start to become more businesslike and the focus will move toward eating rather than playing. By the time they are one year of age, most babies have transitioned naturally to eating purposefully at mealtimes and may already have begun to reduce their need for human milk or formula.

Having scheduled and consistent mealtimes helps babies become aware of their hunger and of the role of food in satisfying it. The most important task for the parent is to make food available at regular times and to respect their baby when she shows them she's done. Pushing babies to eat more than they want can lead to battles over food, or to the overriding of their natural sensation of fullness. Neither of these outcomes is conducive to a healthy long-term relationship with food. For babies to be able to eat when they're hungry and stop when they're full is especially important in populations that are at risk for being overweight, such as babies with Down syndrome, but all babies deserve to have their appetite respected.

ADIEL'S STORY

Jill's account

ADIEL'S HISTORY

Adiel is his parents' third child. His mom is a pediatric nurse. Adiel was diagnosed prenatally with Noonan syndrome and chylothorax (fluid in the outer lining of the lungs). He was born by Cesarean section at 37 weeks, weighing 4 pounds 8 ounces, and remained in the neonatal intensive care unit (NICU) for five weeks. The chylothorax meant he needed a special formula, which he was given via nasogastric tube for most of his NICU stay because his breathing was too rapid to allow oral feedings. He underwent surgery to correct the chylothorax when he was 3 weeks old and, once recovered, was able to begin bottle feeding. One week after the surgery he was having all his feeds by bottle, although he wasn't able to transition to a regular formula until he was 4 months old.

Babies with Noonan syndrome commonly have feeding difficulties, such as a lack of interest in eating or outright feeding aversion, but Adiel did not appear to have these problems. Indeed, his parents were very pleased with his bottle feeding skills, especially given his initial medical challenges and the weeks of nasogastric tube feedings. Following the advice she had been given when her older children were babies, his mom began offering him solid foods by spoon when he was 4 months old. However, he would gag on them and then vomit forcefully. She and his dad tried pureed baby food, chunkier baby food, and pieces of real food, but the same thing happened each time. As a result, and because they were concerned about weight loss, they stopped attempting solids and decided to seek help. Having had two sons who had taken to spoon feeding easily and then moved on to feeding themselves, they wanted to be proactive in getting Adiel the feeding support he needed.

ADIEL'S FEEDING THERAPY INTERVENTION AND PROGRESS

I first evaluated Adiel when he was just 6 months old. At that point, formula, fortified to 22 calories per ounce, was his primary source of nutrition. Prior to our (virtual) meeting, his mom had purchased some items that I had recommended, including some flat-headed spoons and a silicone feeder, so we were all set to implement ABLW. At our first session, I noticed immediately that Adiel's shoulders were below the high chair tray, making it difficult for him to use his arms. I watched him being offered a carrot puree by spoon and immediately turning away from it, although he was happy to accept the spoon when it had no food on it. I suggested his mom try strips of celery and toast and he readily brought them to his mouth to gnaw on, with no signs of aversion. He also gnawed on a silicone feeder filled with avocado, although he then used his tongue to eject what came out of it.

Following this initial consultation, I made several therapy recommendations. First was an insert for the high chair, to raise Adiel up and improve his sitting position. I also suggested including him in family mealtimes, so that he could see others eating and be inspired to copy them. I advocated responsive feeding, in which Adiel's "no" would be respected, and giving him a bottle feed to calm him before putting him in his high chair. I encouraged a focus on handheld foods, such as popsicles, and strips of food for self-feeding, as well as spoons pre-loaded with table-food mashes and the use of a silicone feeder. I persuaded Adiel's parents to stop trying to spoon feed him and instead to work on making mealtimes pleasant and supporting him to feed himself. Alongside this, I recommended that they offer him teething toys and a silicone chew, for discriminative mouthing and chewing practice outside of mealtimes.

Adiel's mom ran with my recommendations. She purchased an insert for Adiel's chair and started offering him table foods instead of purees. He was able to explore foods such as pizza crust, a strip of brisket, a piece of banana with the peel trimmed back (see photo 52), fish sticks, and chicken strips. When he showed signs of trying to overstuff his mouth she would grade his bite size by positioning her finger partway along each strip. He quickly began to demonstrate greatly improved chewing skills and started to pick up food mashes, like mashed potatoes, with his hand. He was also learning to bite and pull on resistive food strips, and to gnaw on large foods, such as a partially peeled kiwi fruit.

Between the ages of 6 and 9 months, Adiel's mom reported a huge change in his interest in, and acceptance of, food. She felt that the seating adaptation played a significant part, in that improving his postural stability made him better able to feed himself. It was also clear that he found self-feeding preferable to being fed by spoon. By 11 months, Adiel was drinking independently from a straw and picking up small food pieces, although he did better when the pieces were offered on his mom or dad's palm than when they were placed on his high chair tray. For extra chewing practice, we started therapeutic fork feeding (see page 204), as well as frozen straws. We helped him avoid overstuffing his mouth by using verbal reminders, or by putting less food in front of him at once. We also encouraged him to practice taking graded bites of large foods, like a peeled pear.

By 13 months, Adiel no longer required my input. He had made incredible strides with his skills and was now feeding himself with a large variety of table foods. He was becoming slightly more selective about what he liked but still ate pretty much everything his parents and brothers were eating. He could pick up and chew small pieces, take bites of foods like pizza, toast, and fresh apricots, and drink from a straw cup. Solid food was now his primary source of nutrition and his mom was slowly weaning him from the bottle onto a cup for his remaining milk feeds.

DISCUSSION

Adiel's feeding skills underwent a very rapid transformation. With an adjustment to his seating and the adoption of baby-led and responsive feeding techniques, he quickly learned to feed himself and began to enjoy food. From the ages of 6 to 13 months, in just seven feeding therapy sessions, he went from being spoon fed and projectile vomiting to eating table foods of all sizes, shapes, and textures—and mealtimes were transformed from extremely stressful to joyous. As a bonus, his previously poor weight gain also improved significantly. In retrospect, his mom felt that 4 months was too young to have introduced him to solid foods and that 6 months gave him a better chance to be an active participant in the process.

Adiel's mom's perspective

Adiel is our third child, so we thought introducing solids would be easy and fun, just like it was for our other two children. Who doesn't love seeing a baby covered in mashed carrots or peas? This would be the first time that we were surprised during our feeding journey, and not in a good way. At 4 months exactly, I set him up in his bouncy seat on our dining room table and shoved some sweet potato baby food into his mouth. He initially moved his tongue around it, then started coughing. Then he started gagging. And then he projectile vomited sweet potato–tinged throw-up all over himself and the bouncy seat. I repeated this process a few times over the next several weeks, telling myself maybe he wasn't ready last time and this time would be different. Once he passed the 6-month mark and was still projectile vomiting from solids, I decided to take some action.

Adiel was prenatally diagnosed with a genetic disorder called Noonan syndrome, and by the time he was born, we were armed with tremendous knowledge and a Facebook group where we could hear from other parents. We knew feeding difficulties are one of the hallmarks of Noonan syndrome and that most babies need to be tube fed during the first year of life. Since Adiel had sailed through bottle feeding with no difficulties, this bump with solids put us out of our depth. I frantically posted in a local group asking for feeding therapy recommendations for infants, and we were connected with Jill. Before our first session, she sent me a list of links for equipment—spoons that looked like teethers and teethers shaped like Ps. The night before our first session, just to try out the flat-headed pre-spoon, I dipped it in the trusty sweet potato baby food and gave it to Adiel. He took it, put it in his mouth, and I sat there waiting for him to throw up. But he didn't. It was the first time we had ever successfully given him solid food. The anxiety I was harboring about solids palpably lifted, and I couldn't wait to learn more about how best to feed him.

Adapted baby-led weaning put Adiel fully in control of his solid food intake. I couldn't believe that a baby was capable of regulating his nutrition and eating foods that most parents would never dream of feeding to an infant. Jill reassured me time and again that the amount of food he was eating was not the point; rather, we were building a positive relationship with food. The absolute most surprising aspect of this journey is realizing that if I could let go and put my child in control of his food, even at the age of 6 months, he knew how to eat. My using a spoon to shovel baby food into his mouth was not the right direction for him, but if I let him hold a giant bone-in rib bigger than his head? He dug right in. If Adiel was able to hold a food, he was able to bring it to his mouth, and eating became one of his favorite activities. Our mealtimes were fun again, laughing at our tiny baby gnawing on a whole chicken leg or putting his face directly into his bowl of yogurt to eat it more efficiently.

Adiel is now a very active 18-month-old. While some meals are still a struggle, we are confident that he knows what he needs for his body, because his foundation with food is so strong. Sure, we get frustrated when we put him in his high chair and he takes one bite and then signs "All done." Or when he's reaching for a food and crying like he really wants it, but then throws it on the floor without even tasting it. Sometimes he skips meals entirely, and then wants seconds—or thirds—at dinner. There are challenges with toddlers regardless of how they eat; that's no surprise. But trusting Adiel's ability to consistently feed himself and regulate his intake without our hovering and intervening has been the most surprising of all.

7

.....

Foods for Learning

For babies who are learning to eat using their hands, the size, shape, and texture of a piece of food is at least as important as its color and flavor. Different textures demand varied chewing skills and provide new types of reward and feedback, while a diversity of shapes and sizes encourages manual dexterity, as well as practice at biting, chewing, and jaw and bite grading (see chapter 3).

In ABLW, foods and drinks are selected for the eating challenges they offer and are used therapeutically, with the aim of both enhancing the baby's current abilities and facilitating, or laying the groundwork for, the next more complicated skill. In contrast to what happens when babies are spoon fed, ABLW introduces large pieces of food from the outset, leading to smaller pieces as the baby's dexterity and oral skills improve, then incorporating bigger foods again as he learns to cope with more complex shapes and textures. This big-small-big principle is one of the aspects of ABLW that many people struggle to understand—until they see it in action.

This chapter describes how to choose and prepare foods and drinks for babies who need extra support with eating, in order to promote learning and ensure safety. Examples of suitable foods in the various formats can be found in Table 2, on page 158, and in the photo insert. But we begin with a look at the nutritional content of family meals.

Preparing family meals

Exactly how each baby transitions to solid foods using an adapted BLW approach will depend on his individual challenges and skills (including any special dietary needs) but the day-to-day choice of foods rests with his parents or other caregivers. Home-cooked foods are generally more nutrient-dense than store-bought baby foods, while minimizing packaging and factory processes that are harmful to the environment. They also offer a wider variety of textures and more calories with less volume, which is especially helpful for babies who struggle with weight gain. Ideally, the foods offered will be those the rest of the household are eating, so it may be helpful to review the family diet in advance of starting ABLW, to allow time for adjustments to be made. However, as a basic principle, if the food can be prepared appropriately to the baby's abilities, and provided ingredients that babies should not have are avoided (see "Foods to avoid," page 157), he can be given the chance to try whatever the family is eating.

When I first saw ABLW in action I was struck by how responsive the parents were to their toddlers, by the independence of the toddlers themselves, and by the variety of foods they were eating at a much earlier age.

Lori Overland, speech-language pathologist

Foods to avoid

The main foods to avoid in your baby's first year are

- ultra-processed foods and those with added salt, sugar, and artificial additives (but note some snack foods may be useful for working on specific feeding skills)
- animal milks offered as a drink (but okay as yogurt, in cooking, or with cereal)
- soy milk (which contains high levels of aluminum and plant estrogens)
- rice milk (which contains arsenic and should be avoided until age 5 years)
- caffeinated and/or sugar-sweetened beverages
- caffeinated foods, such as chocolate
- fruit and vegetable juices
- honey (which can cause botulism)
- unpasteurized milk products and mold-ripened cheeses
- undercooked, unpasteurized eggs
- uncooked and lightly cooked seafood
- shark, swordfish, and marlin (which can contain high levels of pollutants)
- raw bran and bran products (which contain too much fiber)

Check the current Centers for Disease Control and Prevention (CDC) guidelines for up-to-date information.[1]

TABLE 2. FOODS TO ENCOURAGE DEVELOPMENT OF FEEDING SKILLS

TYPE OF FOOD	DESCRIPTION	PURPOSE	
Starter strips and teethers *	Firm 2–3-inch strips or sticks that cannot be bitten through or broken/snapped; ½–1 inch diameter, to match baby's grasp.	Hand-to-mouth movements Eye-hand coordination Cheek contraction Lip closure	Tongue tip mobility Sensory exposure: touch, smell, and taste Reduce sensitivity of gag reflex
	Larger, nonedible food items.	Jaw grading and strength Tongue lateralization	Build oral sensory awareness and promote mouth mapping
Purees and spreadables	Foods of a smooth consistency, ranging from almost liquid through viscous to thick (not flowing), which require no chewing.	Hand-to-mouth movements Eye-hand coordination	Raking grasp Index finger isolation
	(Used with bridge device or dipper, or for hand-to-mouth or finger-to-mouth self-feeding.)	Cheek contraction Lip closure Jaw grading and strength	Tongue tip mobility Sensory exposure: touch, smell, and taste
Mashes	Foods of a coarser consistency than purees, mashed with a masher or fork and requiring minimal chewing.	Hand-to-mouth movements Eye-hand coordination Fine motor skills, such as raking Cheek contraction	Lip closure Tongue tip mobility Practice at moving gaze downward Sensory exposure: touch, smell, and taste
Large foods	Foods that need to be held with two hands and gnawed.	Hand-to-mouth movements Eye-hand coordination Two-handed hold with midline orientation Cheek contraction Lip closure	Gnawing and "shaving" Biting and chewing Jaw grading Tongue lateralization Upper body strength
Soft solids	Pieces, strips, or spears that are moist and easily squished and require minimal chewing.	Hand-to-mouth movements Practice at moving gaze downward Fine motor skills, including pincer grasp Cheek contraction	Lip closure Biting and chewing Jaw grading, stability and strength Tongue lateralization Sensory exposure: touch, smell, and tas

* In adapted BLW, these foods are used for chewing and gnawing practice and to build jaw strength. Some are reintroduced as firm foods for eating once the baby's chewing skills are more refined.

EXAMPLES		IDDSI LEVEL**
Raw carrot (cut flat) Celery stick Kale stalk/rib Romaine lettuce rib	Raw bell pepper Steak Pizza crust	7 (regular solid)
Mango pit (stripped) Meat rib bone (stripped)	Chicken drumstick (stripped) Corn cob (stripped)	N/A
Applesauce Yogurt Pudding	Stage 1 and 2 commercial baby foods	4 (puree)
Pureed avocado Pureed banana Pureed sweet potato Pureed potato Pureed pumpkin	Cream cheese Hummus Thinned nut butters Pureed refried beans	
Cooked root vegetables, such as carrot, potato, sweet potato Avocado Butternut squash	Scrambled eggs Composite meals (e.g., beans mashed with avocado and rice)	5 (fork mash)
Mango pit (with some flesh on) Large strawberry Whole pear (with some peel left on) Kiwi or apricot (partially exposed)	Kiwi disc (cut across, not lengthwise) Peach or nectarine (partially exposed) Piece of banana, with skin cut down Corn on cob disc	7 (regular solid)
Avocado Banana Roasted sweet potato Roasted bell pepper	Very ripe papaya Cooked root vegetables, such as carrot, potato, rutabaga	5 (fork mash)

**International Dysphagia Diet Standardisation Initiative: iddsi.org/framework

TABLE 2. FOODS TO ENCOURAGE DEVELOPMENT OF FEEDING SKILLS (cont.)

TYPE OF FOOD	DESCRIPTION	PURPOSE	
Meltable solids	Crunchy foods that dissolve rapidly in contact with saliva. Whole cracker, piece, or strip.	Hand-to-mouth movements Eye-hand coordination Practice at moving gaze downward Cheek contraction Lip closure	Biting and chewing Jaw grading Tongue lateralization Tongue tip mobility Sensory exposure: touch, smell and tas
Resistive food strips	Strips of foods with "stretchy" quality that require biting and pulling.	Hand-to-mouth movements Cheek contraction Lip closure Biting and chewing	Jaw grading, stability and strength Tongue lateralization Tongue tip mobility
Small food pieces	Small pieces of regular-shaped soft solids that can be put into the mouth whole with fingers or from a fork. May be soft, crunchy, or firm Amount of refined chewing required is dependent on type of piece	Eye-hand coordination Practice at moving gaze downward Fine motor skills, including raking and pincer grasp Cheek Contraction	Lip Closure Biting and chewing Jaw grading, stability, and strength Tongue lateralization Tongue tip mobility
Firmer foods	Firmer strips, spears, and more advanced shapes that require chewing before swallowing.	Hand-to-mouth movements Fine motor skills, including pincer grasp Cheek contraction Lip closure Biting and chewing	Jaw grading, stability, and strength Tongue lateralization Tongue tip mobility Practice at moving gaze downward
Mixed textures	Blend of two or more textures in one dish.	Hand-to-mouth movements Eye-hand coordination Fine motor skills, including pincer grasp Cheek contraction Lip closure Biting and chewing	Jaw grading Tongue lateralization Tongue tip mobility Sensory exposure: touch, smell, and taste Practice at gazing downward

EXAMPLES			IDDSI LEVEL*
Commercial dissolvable puffs and crackers Some freeze-dried fruits			6 (bite-size solid)
Toasted bread Processed cheese (string or slice) Tortilla wrap Waffle	Pancake Steak Cooked asparagus stalk Segment of orange (with membrane removed)		7 (regular solid)
Avocado Banana Kiwi fruit Pasta pieces Potato Roasted red peppers Raspberries Tofu	Egg Steamed carrot Soft cheese (e.g., fresh mozzarella) Puffs Commercial breakfast cereal Peas (soft and squashed)	Blueberries (soft and crushed) Beans Grapes (halved or quartered lengthwise) Chicken Corn kernels	5 (fork mash)/ 6 (bite-size solid)/ 7 (regular solid)
Strawberries Roasted zucchini Cereal bars (softer brands) Blueberries (soft and crushed) Pasta pieces Cucumber	Broccoli floret Cheese strip (cut from block) Sweet potato fries Toast Fish Chicken		6 (bite-size solid)/ 7 (regular solid), depending on how they are cut/prepared
Soups Casseroles Lasagna Stage 3 commercial baby foods	Cereal with milk Smooth food with pieces, like yogurt with pieces of fruit		5 (fork mash)/ 6 (bite-size solid)/ 7 (regular solid), mixed, as appropriate, with 0 (thin liquid)

First foods do not have to be bland. Babies who are hyper-sensitive to flavors tend to prefer simple tastes, but others may enjoy quite spicy foods. Plus, herbs and spices are a great way to add flavor to family meals without using salt. Babies who have been fed using hydrolysate formulas will have become accustomed to a bitter taste and may be surprisingly receptive to foods such as artichoke and brussels sprouts. For adults and babies alike, a varied diet helps to ensure good nutrition. The more colorful the meal, and the greater the number of flavors it contains, the more likely it is to include all the macro- and micronutrients needed. Variety is also important for stimulat-ing interest in food and for enhancing eating pleasure.

The wider the range of foods to which a baby is exposed in the first months of complementary feeding, and the more real they are in appearance (as opposed to just being pureed or mashed), the bigger the reference database he will build of linked images, smells, flavors, and textures. This means that, at the point when the visual appearance of food begins to become a key factor in his decisions about what he is willing to eat (around the time he starts walking),[2] fewer foods will appear new. Indeed, babies have been shown to develop food preferences based on the color of the foods they were exposed to most often early on, so the more colorful the better.[3]

The main micronutrient most babies begin to need in addi-tional amounts from 6 months onward is iron. It's therefore important that they are offered foods that are a good source of iron from the outset. (Zinc may also be needed but it tends to be present in the same foods as iron.) Meat is the richest source of iron but using a cast-iron cooking pot or (from 7 months) a

Lucky Iron Fish may help to increase the iron content of other foods. If the start of solid foods needs to be delayed to allow the baby time to develop the necessary foundational skills, it may be appropriate to discuss iron supplementation with his pediatrician or dietitian.

> Why should children with feeding difficulties be limited to bland, mushy foods? They deserve flavorful foods just as much as their peers.
>
> Amy Manojlovski, registered dietitian

Early shapes, sizes, and textures

The presentation of foods in a variety of sizes, shapes, and textures from the outset is a distinguishing feature of both BLW and ABLW. However, while babies whose development follows a typical path are usually able to cope with several different foods at once, the progression through the various formats must be more closely managed for those whose needs are different.

Starter strips and food teethers

A strip or stick of food is a great first shape for a baby to hold because it's easy for him to grasp and will fit neatly between the chewing surfaces of his gums. The ideal length is two to three inches; this allows part of the strip to act as a "handle" inside the baby's hand and the rest to stick out beyond his fist, for him to gnaw on. The strip should be around a half to one inch wide, so that it fills his fist while allowing his hand to close around it fully. This will allow him to pick it up more easily and control it more effectively than if his hand were either too tightly closed or partially open.

Starter strips are not intended for eating. Instead, they allow the baby to experience the taste and texture of real food while practicing the building blocks of chewing through reflexive jaw movements. The repetitive motion of chewing on firm strips on alternating sides of the mouth will increase his jaw strength and may even encourage his teeth to come in earlier. Raw vegetables make great starter strips, especially when cut with flat edges so that they sit effectively between the baby's gums. At this stage, he will not be able to either chew or spit out pieces of food, so, if he is able to bite through raw vegetables, then a food teether, such as a mango pit, is a safer alternative. Luan (page 178) made great progress in chewing using starter strips.

Starter strips and food teethers provide excellent sensory feedback, assisting the process of mouth mapping (see page 64). They are also useful for promoting tongue lateralization as a way of discouraging a persistent tongue thrust (see pages 70 and 131). Early and frequent practice with these foods contributes to the development of both efficient chewing and safe eating. This is especially important for babies with atypical oral motor development, who are inclined to swallow foods before they are sufficiently broken down, creating a concern for choking and poor digestion.

Purees, spreadables, and mashes

While purees and mashed foods are not considered necessary as first foods in regular BLW, they play an important role in the transitional phase that is a distinguishing feature of ABLW. The use of soft, mushy foods allows babies who require an extra level of support with feeding to feed themselves from the outset, rather than needing to be spoon fed.

Purees and mashed foods can be of varying consistencies (see Table 2, page 158). Very thin, semi-liquid purees, such as applesauce, can be used on a (pre-loaded) spoon or in a silicone feeder (see page 190), but they will usually be very messy, as well as being frustrating for the baby. A more viscous texture, like yogurt, may work better. Thin purees can also be drunk via a cup or straw (see page 195), while thicker purees are useful as dips to encourage dexterity and pave the way for utensil use (see "Foods for dipping," page 166). Pureed soft foods, and spreadable family foods like hummus, offer more advanced and interesting textures, as do composite meals, for example, soft brown rice mashed together with beans.

Not all babies will require a transitional phase that includes the use of purees, but those who do will need to be introduced to lumpier foods as early as they can manage them, in order to promote chewing and reduce the chances of longer-term eating difficulties.[4] Coarsely mashed soft foods provide a useful transition for babies who are not yet ready to bite and chew, since they create an awareness of texture variation inside the mouth. They may also help stimulate the tongue to begin to move food to the chewing surfaces. They can be offered initially on a pre-loaded spoon or in a feeder, then placed directly on the high chair tray for the baby to explore and bring to his mouth. This will have the additional advantage of helping him coordinate his movements, first picking up a handful of mash using his whole hand, then gradually, with practice, making smaller and more accurate movements with his fingers, eventually leading to a refined pincer grasp.

Foods for dipping

Dipping is a useful skill that is a precursor to regular use of utensils, promoting manual dexterity as well as the oral skill of lip closure. Spoons can act as dippers, but so, too, can a variety of foods. And, because a food dipper can be held either way up, many babies initially find them easier to manage. Starter strips, stick-shaped meltable solids, and some resistive food strips make great early dippers, while the dip itself can be any type of savory or sweet puree, spreadable food, or soft mash. For example, a strip of cucumber could be used to dip into yogurt. The dipper can be offered pre-loaded, either from the caregiver's hand or sticking up out of the dip for the baby to grasp. Placing the dip within the baby's reach and demonstrating the dipping action will encourage him to copy it.

Initially, the dipper is just a way for the baby to get the dip to his mouth, but as his biting skills develop, he will be able to bite into the dipper itself, so getting a mix of flavors and textures. Indeed, dipping is a neat way to introduce the concept of food combinations, although it's a good idea to ensure that the baby is already familiar with—and likes—both the dipper and the dip before offering them together.

Large foods

A great way to expand a baby's food repertoire and work on chewing skills, graded jaw movements, and bite size is to offer large foods for the baby to gnaw on and shave with his gums or teeth. Large foods have the advantage that they can't easily be stuffed into the mouth whole. In addition, foods that require two hands to hold motivate the baby to practice using both hands together in midline, something that is often particularly difficult for babies with neurodevelopmental issues.

It's helpful if the food is presented in a way that makes it easy to hold; slippery foods can be frustrating, especially for babies who have low muscle tone. A peach, for example, might be left unpeeled but have a channel cut through the center, so the baby can hold the skin on the outside and taste the fleshy middle (see suggestions in photos 28–30). Similarly, a banana can be offered as a three- or four-inch piece with a quarter inch of peel removed or as a chunk loaded onto a small round-handled fork (see photo 53). Round foods, like avocado or kiwi fruit, can be placed in a small ramekin, cup, or jar (or the cap from a feeding bottle) to make them more stable (see Adira, photo 27). Another option is to cut the bottom off the fruit to give it a flat base, then stand it directly on the tray. This not only makes the food easier for the baby to grasp and pick up but also allows him to steady it with his hands and lean forward to gnaw on it.

Medium-size flat shapes that require two hands to hold, such as a disk of kiwi fruit or corn (see Thiago, photo 42) encourage a different grasp and are particularly useful for helping babies learn to grade their bite size. Larger flat foods, like slices of watermelon, and those that need to be bitten into rather than gnawed, such as sandwiches, demand more mature skills, so will not feature until later.

Modeling how to eat

Involving babies in family mealtimes is a key part of BLW, enabling them to observe how others eat and to copy their actions. However, ABLW can involve offering babies foods in shapes and sizes (such as a whole avocado, semi-peeled) that they will not have seen in regular use at the family table. Alternatively, they may be familiar with the presentation of the food but have seen it eaten with utensils, not with fingers—mashed potato, for example. In these situations the caregiver can demonstrate what the baby needs to do by themselves picking up an avocado to gnaw, or by putting their finger in the mash, raking up a small amount and bringing it to their mouth. This is more helpful to the baby than simply placing the food in front of him and expecting him to figure out what to do. It is also a less pressuring approach for babies who are cautious when presented with something new than urging them to "Try it" or "Take a bite."

Soft solid strips

The first true finger foods—for eating, rather than for biting and gnawing—are strips of foods that are firm enough for the baby to hold but soft enough for him to bite into and munch or chew with minimal effort. For some foods, such as avocado, the degree of ripeness is key. The "squish" test (see photo 51) is a useful way to figure this out: If the strip can be held between an adult's thumb and index finger without disintegrating but can also be compressed easily, that's a soft solid consistency.

Like starter strips, soft solid strips need to be cut into stick shapes that allow the baby's fist to close fully around the width of the food, leaving one or two inches sticking out. This is because, even though the intention is for him to eat the food, until he is more experienced and dexterous he will not be able to open his hand voluntarily to get at what's inside. Slippery foods can be made easier to grip by rolling the pieces in fine breadcrumbs, chia seeds, or ground flaxseed, or by leaving some of the peel on. Cutting foods with a crinkle cutter is another way to make them easier to grasp. Photos 55–58 show some examples.

It's likely that when he first begins to handle soft food strips, the baby will squeeze them too hard. This isn't necessarily a problem, since he can still take the food to his mouth and taste it—it will just take time and practice for him to adjust his grip to hold soft foods without squishing them (as Faith is doing in photo 44) and to discover how to take bites. He will likely also want to spend time looking at the food and moving it around on the tray before he picks it up, especially if it's new to him. It may appear as though he's "just" playing with it, but this exploration is an important part of his learning, helping him to anticipate how the food will behave inside his mouth and to recognize the same food the next time he sees it. Once he has developed the ability to take bites out of the food and move the bitten-off pieces from the center of his mouth to the chewing surfaces of his gums, soft solids can become part of his regular food repertoire and he will be ready to attempt more challenging textures.

Meltable solids

Meltable solids are crunchy snack foods, such as puffs, that come in different sizes, shapes, and flavors, and dissolve easily in about ten seconds, once mixed with saliva. While they are not recommended as part of a regular diet for most children because of their ultra-processed nature, they do offer therapeutic benefits for babies with feeding challenges. They also enable the introduction of potential allergens, such as dairy and peanut, in an easily edible form. They therefore have a place within a managed feeding plan. The best options are those that are most nutritionally dense, with a high vitamin and mineral content and few or no artificial additives, so it's worth comparing labels or conferring with a dietitian.

Stick-shaped meltable solids provide useful practice at taking bites off, which helps with jaw strengthening and grading. Their texture encourages the baby to use fine-graded repetitive bites, which are an important part of learning to chew, while their dissolvability means that any pieces that get bitten off present a very low risk of choking. They also tend to behave in a predictable fashion, with a consistent flavor, meaning they may be more acceptable than some other foods to babies who have learned that certain foods are not to be trusted.

As well as being useful for biting at the front of the mouth, meltable solids can be positioned on the lateral surface of the gums to help with sustained chewing and desensitization of the inner surface of the cheeks (to encourage acceptance of lumpier foods). Evan, in photo 67, is demonstrating this. Another feature in their favor is their crunchiness, which gives great sensory feedback. This makes eating them fun for the baby, while increasing his oral sensory awareness; this is especially valuable for babies with low muscle tone. Used in a silicone feeder, they help both the baby and his caregiver to recognize small, even, repetitive chewing movements, based on the sound heard when the baby's chewing is effective.

Resistive strips

Resistive foods, which have a stretchy texture, are perfect for helping to develop jaw strength and sensory perception, as well as coordination of hand and mouth movements. In an effort to bite through the strip, the baby will grip it between his gums and pull his hand away, stretching the piece. At the same time, he will tend to move his tongue to where the food is, encouraging lateral tongue mobility. As his jaw strength and graded control improve, he will be able to maintain his grip until the food tears and a small piece comes off. With practice, he will be able to progress to foods that offer greater resistance.

Moving on: firmer foods and new shapes

As the baby's fine motor and oral skills develop, firmer textures and more advanced shapes can be introduced, along with strips of food that yield pieces that require more refined chewing. A little later still, he will be able to cope with foods that generate dry crumbs, such as breadsticks and cookies. Once he has had plenty of practice at picking up mashes and strips of food from his tray, he will also be ready to move on to small pieces of food that can be put into his mouth whole.

Small food pieces

Small food pieces are great for working on a pincer grasp, as well as on fine chewing skills. The exact size of the pieces to be offered will vary depending on the texture of the food, the baby's current level of dexterity, and his skills at chewing and moving food around inside his mouth. The choice of food should be guided by the baby's feeding therapist, who will know what he can manage safely.

The first small food pieces will usually be soft solids, such as fresh mozzarella or goat cheese, that can be broken down easily with gentle pressure from the baby's gums. These require minimal effort to chew and are less likely to become stuck on his tongue and cause gagging, which could make both him and his caregivers anxious. Small pieces of meltable solids are another option, as they are easy to pick up and dissolve readily. Round, firm foods—like slices of hot dog or whole grapes—should be avoided because they could become lodged in the baby's airway. Peas and blueberries can be squashed to make them safer but they will usually be offered later, since they require a more refined pincer grasp and a higher level of oral skill for safe maneuvering, and they need to be thoroughly chewed before swallowing.

Foods that crumble

When babies are first introduced to foods that are drier, or that crumble or scatter into pieces in their mouth, such as ground meat, they can find them difficult to gather together with their tongue. Mixing the food with something moist, such as yogurt, sour cream, or applesauce, can make the bolus stickier, helping it to stay together and making it less likely that bits will fall out of the baby's mouth or get lost in his cheeks.

Picking up small food pieces and transferring them to the mouth is a complex skill. In typically developing babies it is usually present by 9 months, but because it requires refined movement and control of the thumb and index finger, successful aim into the mouth, and controlled oral manipulation, it can necessitate some modifications for babies who have developmental delay or limited movement. For example, the baby may find it easier, initially, to pick up the piece of food from the caregiver's outstretched hand, halfway between the high chair tray and his mouth, rather than directly from the tray. He may also benefit from the caregiver's supporting his hand from underneath to help him direct the food into his mouth. Avoiding slippery foods will help to reduce frustration.

A baby's initial attempts to pick up small pieces of food from a flat surface usually involve a poking gesture, followed by a raking movement. As he develops greater core strength and stability this will be accompanied by increased muscular control and strength in his hands, allowing him to grip the food with his fingertips rather than his whole hand, and eventually evolving into a true pincer grasp, using just the thumb and index finger. A caregiver can assist the development of the pincer grasp by holding the baby's wrist as he picks up the food. This helps stabilize the wrist, allowing more refined movements of the fingers. The caregiver can also offer the food piece between their own thumb and forefinger, meaning the baby has to use more precise finger movements to take it (see Adira, photo 46). Putting a food piece into a section cut from an egg carton is another way to help babies learn to isolate their finger and thumb to pick up something small. As the

Each baby will master the various sizes, shapes, and textures of food at his own pace and in his own style. Some will progress smoothly and steadily, while others will gain skills in bursts, with long periods of consolidation in between. Given time and plenty of practice, almost all babies will eventually be able to manage a wide range of foods presented in a variety of formats and feed themselves both with their fingers and with utensils.

> Alanna was diagnosed with acid reflux at 4 months old, and by the time she was ready to start solid foods we could see the reflux might make things difficult. Until that point we had never heard of BLW, but putting Alanna in charge of what she would eat seemed like a good idea. My family were very skeptical in the beginning, but when they saw her at 7 months old munching down on a lamb chop, they were blown away. It was not just the beginning of weaning anymore—it was the start of Alanna's relationship with food.
>
> Áine, mother of Alanna, 17 months,
> who had reflux until 15 months

Foods for drinking

In the early months of complementary feeding, babies can continue to get all the fluid they need from either the breast or bottle, but there are advantages to learning the skill of drinking from an open cup—and, later, a straw (see page 82)—especially for babies who face oral motor challenges. Cup drinking is also useful for a baby who has been tube fed for a long period and who may have difficulty breastfeeding or sucking from a bottle. Indeed, some babies who have been tube fed bypass drinking from the breast or bottle and go directly to cup and straw drinking in the latter half of their first year. And then there are babies who simply prefer to have their first tastes of family food in liquid form.

Many babies who are following a program of adapted BLW can take awhile to really begin eating. For some, this may mean there are concerns over weight gain. Offering them fortified or thickened drinks is a useful way to provide extra nutrients and calories while their self-feeding skills catch up. If the baby is under the care of a dietitian, they may recommend ways to further increase calorie intake with the addition of, for example, whipping cream or oils. Blending foods into smoothies is also a great way to introduce allergens like dairy or tahini to the diet of a baby who is not yet able to manage solid versions of those foods.

The first drinks offered by cup will usually be human milk and/or infant formula. Other suitable liquids include purees thinned with human milk or formula, well-blended smoothies, yogurt drinks, and even smooth soups. While some babies cope better with warm feeds, cold fluids will give more sensory feedback, allowing the baby to feel more easily how the milk is behaving in his mouth.[5] For babies who need help to tolerate a wider range of textures, foods offered by cup can be made gradually thicker; soups and smoothies are ideal for this purpose.

Not all babies find it easy to swallow liquids, especially from an open cup. Milk, water, and other fluids behave differently from solids; they are harder to control and can readily escape.

They may spill forward out of the mouth, making drinking tiring, unrewarding, and messy, or backward into the airway, causing coughing and potentially finding their way into the lungs (aspiration). Thin fluids are the most challenging, so thickening them provides a solution (see Theodora's story, page 235). Some commonly used thickeners are oatmeal, pureed foods, and proprietary thickeners. The degree of thickening will be gradually reduced as the baby's oral skills become more refined.

Some babies' swallowing difficulties will appear very early, necessitating thickened bottle feeds, while others may encounter problems when they begin using a cup or straw. The results of a swallowing assessment—VFSS or FEES (see page 100)—will determine whether and to what degree thickening is necessary, based on the IDDSI international framework.[6] Table 2, on page 158, shows how the types of foods and fluids used in ABLW fit with the IDDSI classification. A therapist can work on improving the baby's ability to manage liquids safely by cautiously introducing small amounts that are slightly thinner than those he is used to. After some practice, a repeat VFSS or FEES will help to determine whether this thinner consistency can now be used for all his drinks.

LUAN'S STORY

Jill's account

LUAN'S HISTORY

Luan is his parents' second child. He was born at 36 weeks' gestation and was quickly noted to have both esophageal atresia and anal atresia as well as only three fingers and a thumb on his left hand. Esophageal atresia is a condition in which the upper and lower parts of the esophagus are separated, each having a blind end or pouch. This means that food is unable to pass from the mouth to the stomach. Anal atresia refers to an anal opening that is either absent or not properly formed, which causes difficulty in stooling.

Luan had initial surgery for his esophageal atresia when he was 1 day old. Three weeks later, he was able to receive 5 milliliters of his mom's milk orally every four hours. He left the hospital at 2 months, at which point he was taking most of his feedings by bottle, although his mom was able to practice breastfeeding with him for a few days before he was discharged. Once at home, she slowly increased the amount of breastfeeding until he transitioned to exclusive breastfeeding at 4 months old. He continued to breastfeed until he was 11 months, receiving bottles only when his mom was at work. At 8 months, he underwent a surgical correction of the anal atresia.

LUAN'S FEEDING THERAPY INTERVENTION AND PROGRESS

Luan and his family live in Switzerland. His parents had followed BLW with their first child and were interested in doing the same with Luan—they just weren't sure that his diagnoses would allow it. His mom reached out to Gill via email in March 2021, and Gill asked me if I could help. I was happy to agree.

Luan, his mom, and I met virtually for the first time when he was 7 months old, and I was able to observe him and learn about his medical history. At the conclusion of that meeting I recommended some items for his parents to buy to help him transition to self-feeding, namely a high chair with an adjustable footrest, flat spoons for pre-loading, and a silicone feeder to help with hand-to-mouth and chewing skills. At this point, Luan was sitting up securely and appeared ready to start eating. According to his mom, there were no specific medical issues at that time that precluded him from feeding himself. However, the repair to his esophagus meant that it was shortened and lacked elasticity. We therefore agreed it would be preferable for him to start with soft mashes rather than strips of food, to allow his chewing skills time to mature. After our meeting, Luan's parents duly began offering him mashed banana on a pre-loaded spoon, and starter food strips for chewing practice. They also tried him with open-cup drinking. They reported that "He likes eating!"

Two weeks later, Luan, his mom, and I met again virtually. During this session, he was seated on her lap and was feeding himself pre-loaded spoonfuls of a home-prepared soft mash of sweet potato, apple, carrot, and quinoa. He managed to take bites from a steamed carrot strip but tended to push the pieces out with his tongue because he wasn't yet able to move them to the side of his mouth for chewing. He gnawed on a whole banana and a cantaloupe wedge, took bites of banana spears, and was able to pick up mashed banana from the table and get it to his mouth with his hand. He also took assisted sips of a thinned smooth puree, putting both hands on the cup. Luan's esophagus was functioning well, but maximizing his ability to break down each mouthful would enable food to pass more easily into his stomach. I therefore recommended that he continue with firm starter strips, food teethers, and pre-loaded spoons and practice with small graded bites from soft solid strips, with the addition of frozen straws to further encourage biting and chewing.

Luan's mom and I kept in contact sporadically via email for the next seven months, and Luan continued to progress with his ABLW journey. When he was 13 months old we had another virtual consultation, by which time he was reportedly eating everything the family was eating—including pizza and sushi—which his parents were cutting into small pieces. He was especially fond of bread, which his mom would soften with liquids. I saw him eating rice, and bread soaked in a little herbal tea, using a pincer grasp to pick it up. I was also able to watch him eating a carrot soup, unaided, using a spoon, and drinking thin liquids from an open cup.

Luan had become accustomed to food in small pieces and, when faced with a firm strip of food, attempted to stuff the whole of it into his mouth rather than "bite and pull." I suggested that he be introduced to resistive strips of cheese and bread, to increase his jaw strength and help him gauge how big a bite to take from larger pieces of food. I also recommended encouraging him to gnaw on large foods, such as a whole peeled pear, to stimulate graded jaw movement and to continue with starter food strips and frozen straws.

I am no longer seeing Luan regularly but his mom continues to implement my suggestions and has sent me videos to show his progress. At 15 months, he is rapidly catching up with his peers. He still finds strips difficult to manage without overstuffing but is already discovering how to take bites from larger foods. He is quite adept at using a spoon and at drinking from an open cup, and he uses both hands equally to feed himself.

DISCUSSION

Luan's medical team initially doubted that he could breastfeed or transition to solid foods with baby-led weaning because of his diagnosis. I felt they looked at his limitations rather than his skills and adjusted their expectations accordingly. His mom later told me that his surgeon was impressed and amazed with Luan's eating and wanted to know "How did you do this?" By observing Luan's skill level and selecting food shapes, textures, and therapeutic techniques, I was able to coach his mom safely through the ABLW process, but it was her perseverance and advocacy that enabled him to breastfeed and transition to solids in a baby-led way, just like his brother.

Luan's mom's perspective

Luan was born at 36 weeks. In his first two months, he was living in the neonatal intensive care unit and had already overcome several vital operations (trachea and esophagus, intestine, and heart). Initially, he had to stay in bed to limit movement, and was not given any oral nutrition until the surgical scar had healed. After three weeks, he was allowed to drink 5 milliliters of my milk every four hours (first by syringe and then by bottle). This amount was increased every day. What he could not drink was given to him through the stomach tube. Since Luan's weight was rather low, the staff added formula to my milk to increase the calorie content.

A few days before Luan could go home, I started breastfeeding him twice a day. Since he was only allowed to drink every four hours and was therefore constantly hungry, this was a challenge. Unfortunately, my husband and I did not succeed in convincing the doctors to feed Luan according to his needs and not according to a strict schedule. A few times, a hospital speech therapist visited Luan and gave us some advice, for example, about how to pace his feedings. When we finally got home, I was able to breastfeed him following his needs. Gradually, the amount of supplementary feedings was reduced and natural breastfeeding took over. This led to his gaining more weight. He also became more even-tempered because he could breastfeed whenever he wanted, instead of having to wait four hours between feeds, as prescribed by the doctor.

We had successfully practiced BLW with our firstborn child, so when Luan was about 6 months old, we looked for people who had experience with BLW with disabled babies. Luan's surgeon was not familiar with the BLW method, and knowing Luan's medical history, he was skeptical about this approach. As we could not find a BLW expert for disabled children in German-speaking countries, we turned to Gill Rapley, and she referred us to Jill Rabin. Despite Luan's medical limitations, Jill was very optimistic and confident that BLW was possible for him, and she encouraged us to go ahead.

Through several video consultations, Jill got to know Luan and me and she was able to give us helpful advice for implementing adapted BLW. For example, she recommended using a special spoon, and thickening liquids to a nectar consistency (IDDSI level 2) to make them easier for Luan to drink without choking. She also advised us which foods were better to encourage chewing, and how to increase the calorie content of his meals by adding peas or avocados. It was great to see how much Luan enjoyed sitting in his high chair, participating in family meals, and how quickly his eating skills progressed. In addition, he made significant progress in his fine motor skills through feeding himself, often choosing to eat with his disabled hand even though the other hand functions normally.

Luan ate the same food as we did, with the only exception that the consistency of his meals was sometimes slightly adjusted, for example, by adding cereal to his soup, softening the crust of his pizza, or giving him salad as a smoothie. He was drinking herbal tea, water, or homemade fruit juices with an open cup. Every few weeks, he was examined by his surgeon, who was very surprised at how well Luan gained weight (he went from underweight to normal weight in an unexpectedly short time). He was always curious about how Luan was doing with ABLW but couldn't quite figure out the method. For example, he found it strange that a one-year-old child liked to eat sushi and had no problems eating noodle soup by himself. Luan's success with eating encouraged us that we had made the right decision to use a baby-led approach, despite his diagnosis.

8

.....

Transitioning to Solids with ABLW

Adapted BLW differs from regular BLW primarily in the existence of a transitional phase, during which the baby is supported as she develops the skills she needs to feed herself. This transitional phase is characterized by a variety of therapeutic interventions, including facilitation and the use of bridge devices, as well as specific feeding techniques and the use of cups and straws. This chapter describes these interventions and suggests how, with the support of a qualified feeding therapist, they may form part of an individual baby's journey to independent self-feeding. We begin, however, with the importance of gaining a baby's permission and how to go about this.

Gaining permission

A fundamental element of both pre-feeding exercises (described in chapter 5) and therapeutic feeding interventions is the need to be responsive to the baby and gain her voluntary cooperation with what is being asked of her—not least because this may include the use of techniques and devices that are not of her choosing.

The concept of permission is encapsulated in the Get Permission Approach developed by occupational therapist Marsha Dunn Klein.[1] Klein explains this as being "rooted in the principles of responsive feeding and actively promot[ing] a child's autonomy while fostering connection, trust, and consistent communication between the child and caregiver."[2] Using this approach with spoon feeding, the caregiver presents the food at the baby's mouth and waits for her to indicate her permission by leaning toward the food (defined as a "positive tilt") and/or opening her mouth to receive it. ABLW applies this same principle to supported self-feeding.

Babies exhibit a variety of behaviors around mealtime to indicate they are interested in eating or tasting a food. They may gaze at the food their parent is eating or holding in their hand; they may even reach for it. They may make lip-smacking sounds or verbally fuss, to indicate that they want to join in when others are eating. These behaviors are relatively easy to interpret, since the baby initiates them. The situation is different when the caregiver or therapist is seeking to engage the baby's interest: In this case it's up to the adult to pose the question "May I?" or "Would you like to?," using words and simple non-threatening gestures, then wait and watch for a positive response from the baby. Gaining permission may require repeated attempts and a lot of time and patience but the trust it builds is key to more rapid and rewarding progress later.

In ABLW, the need to gain permission starts well before the food arrives at the baby's mouth. For example, when assisting a baby who is not yet able to pick up a piece of food, the parent or therapist will first offer a starter strip by touching it to the baby's hand. If she opens her fist, she is granting permission for them to present it to her palm. Provided there is no resistance to gentle pressure on the back of her fingers, she can be helped to close her fist around it. The next step will be to apply similar pressure to move her hand to her mouth, looking for her to either allow the movement or tense her arm muscles to resist it. Only when the baby has given her permission for the food to be brought to her lips will the caregiver be looking for her to open her mouth.

Caregivers need to be equally alert to avoidant behaviors. These may be obvious; for example, a baby who is batting food away, turning her head, crying, gagging, or vomiting— or resisting being put in her high chair in the first place—is giving a very clear message. Other signals, though, will be more subtle. Some less-than-obvious examples would be, for a younger baby, yawning during the meal, being easily distracted, or repeatedly trying to engage with her parent rather than focusing on the food. For an older baby, playing excessively with the food would indicate a wish to avoid eating. These are referred to as "blocking" behaviors.

> In my practice I see so many babies who have never
> been asked to give their permission or be partners when
> things are done TO them. No wonder they don't want to
> cooperate!
>
> Marsha Dunn Klein, occupational therapist and founder
> of the Get Permission Institute

A focus on gaining permission is particularly important for babies whose feeding challenges stem from a neuromotor disorder, since they are likely to need an extended transitional phase, involving a large degree of facilitation and targeted exercises. For example, the therapist may seek to place a small piece of a soft solid food on the molar area of the baby's gums to encourage chewing, or position a flat-headed spoon, pre-loaded with puree, on the baby's lower lip to encourage her to use her upper lip in isolation to remove the food. The baby will be much happier to repeat these exercises if her permission is always sought.

Permission is especially crucial for babies with feeding aversion because they are already anxious and apprehensive when it comes to eating. Unfortunately, it is all too easy for the adults involved to overlook this fundamental requirement because of other concerns. For example, many parents of babies with feeding challenges are anxious about their baby's weight gain. They may be worried that she isn't taking in enough volume or find themselves under pressure from her health care provider or a family member to encourage her to eat more. This can make it difficult for them to ask their baby's permission, for fear she will refuse. Unfortunately, ignoring or overriding a baby's cues is apt to increase her sense of being under pressure and make it even more likely she will try to avoid eating.

Facilitation

Facilitation is a technique commonly employed as part of ABLW. It acts as a scaffold to enable the baby to be in charge of her own eating even though she doesn't yet have the skills to feed herself. Facilitation is not the same as helping, even though it may look like it from the outside. It requires the caregiver to be fully responsive to the baby's subtlest signals and to gain her permission at every stage. Although initially the baby and the caregiver will hold the food together, the caregiver won't attempt to steer the baby's movements or place anything in her mouth without first obtaining her permission. The aim is for the caregiver's input to be reduced over time, allowing the baby to feed herself unaided as soon as she is able. The result is maximum autonomy and agency for the baby, from the very beginning.

Facilitation allows babies who are not yet able to bring food to their mouth to experience oral sensations and start to practice the skills needed for effective eating. It also enables those who have a physical disability that would otherwise make self-feeding very difficult or impossible, for example, an absence of fingers, to feed themselves. The following box, "Responsive facilitation," illustrates what facilitation looks like with a starter food strip, but the technique is much the same for a bridge device or straw cup.

Responsive facilitation

Many babies following ABLW need support to get food to their mouth, at least initially. These are the steps to facilitation:

- First, make sure the baby is seated well and comfortably and is not either sleepy or very hungry. (It's never easy to learn a new skill when you're tired or unhappy.)

- Hold out the strip of food in midline, at eye level, ensuring that the baby has a neutral head position, and see if she can grasp it independently. If she has difficulty, wait for her permission to place it in her hand, then provide support by holding her arm at the wrist with one of your hands, and the bottom of the food strip with the other.

- Wait for the baby to indicate interest in the food by looking at it, leaning forward toward it, and/or opening her mouth for it.

- Guide the baby's hand to her mouth, aiming the strip toward the surface of her lower gum, roughly at the point where the first molar will erupt, so that she can gnaw on it.

- Allow her to practice chewing and gnawing and to explore the food with her tongue, maintaining the support as necessary to keep the food inside her mouth.

- After a while, and with the baby's permission, help her to withdraw the food and present it to the opposite gum, so that she develops equal coordination and strength on both sides of her mouth.

- If any resistance is sensed in the baby's arm or hand at any point, or if she moves her head backward or to the side, relax your hold and wait for her to indicate what she wants to do.

Bridge Devices

Bridge devices are feeding utensils that provide babies facing feeding challenges with additional support during the transition to full self-feeding. They do this by enabling the baby to bring food to her mouth more easily, thereby making the process less laborious and increasing the chances that at least some of the food will be eaten. They can also be helpful for babies with sensory issues, who aren't yet ready to touch food with their fingers or hands. Bridge devices consist of pre-loaded spoons, silicone and netted feeders, food popsicles, and frozen straws. They are used in a variety of overlapping ways in order to promote specific skills.

Pre-loaded spoons

A pre-loaded spoon is one that is loaded (and reloaded) by the caregiver, then offered to the baby to hold and bring to her mouth herself. Pre-loaded spoons have a minor role in regular BLW, to enable babies who can't yet manage a spoon for themselves to eat sloppy foods. However, they are a key feature of adapted BLW as a way of helping babies who have motor challenges, or a tactile aversion, to bring food to their mouth. A soft spoon can also offer a degree of chewing practice, much like a starter food strip, although it's less useful in this respect than a silicone feeder.

It's important that the spoon is one designed for a baby to manipulate: The handle should be short and shaped so as to be easily graspable, while the bowl should be small and, ideally, flat or very shallow. A flat-headed dipper spoon, or pre-spoon as used by Eva and Owen in photos 18 and 19 and Ava in photo 48, requires less effort and a less-refined technique than a conventional spoon with a deep bowl, making it easier for the baby to remove the food. It is therefore less frustrating and more rewarding for the novice self-feeder to use.

Initially, the spoon can be offered for the baby to grasp from the caregiver's hand. In this case it will need to be presented in a vertical upright position, rather than in the position that adults use for scooping from a bowl. Alternatively, if this will be difficult for the baby, the spoon can be put directly into her hand. If necessary, gentle facilitation can be used to help guide the spoon, with the caregiver holding the baby's wrist with one hand and steadying the bottom of the spoon handle with the other. As the baby grows, and if pre-loaded spoons continue to be needed, she can progress to a shallow-bowled spoon with a longer handle.

Pre-loading of spoons will commonly begin with a thin puree, to reduce the risk that the baby will gag on the novel texture. This will be followed by something more viscous, then more textured mashes, and eventually combination mashes. While some gagging is normal when babies are learning to eat (see page 71), it is important that, for babies with neurodevelopmental or sensory issues or a history of aversion, their early eating experiences don't present too much of a challenge. Beginning with smooth foods and changing the texture gradually increases the likelihood that the baby's attempts to eat will be rewarding and give her time to desensitize before tackling more demanding textures. As she adjusts to managing food in her mouth, the lumpiness of the food offered can be gradually increased. So, a typical progression might be: applesauce → yogurt → hummus → beans mashed with soft rice.

Silicone and netted feeders

A feeder is a device that can be used either in parallel with, or in place of, a pre-loaded spoon. The advantage of a feeder is that, in addition to helping the baby get food to her mouth, it allows her to work on graded chewing and gnawing. Feeders can also be useful for resistive chewing practice, in which the baby grips the feeder with her gums while pulling with her hand, in the same way as she might do with a strip of steak or toast. They are also helpful for babies with neurodevelopmental issues, who are often able to take a bite from a piece of food but struggle to manage and chew the bitten-off part; using a feeder avoids this.

Another situation in which a feeder can be useful is when a parent or other caregiver is unusually fearful of their baby's choking. In this case the feeder allows the baby a degree of autonomy and the chance to practice important skills, while reducing stress for the parent. Once they are more comfortable with the baby's abilities the feeder can be discarded. A feeder is also an option for occasional use by caregivers who struggle to cope with mess, or in a daycare situation where the staff may not be confident to implement BLW. In general, though, feeders should be considered a therapeutic device rather than a regular way for babies who do not need this support to feed themselves.

There are many different styles of feeder. All of them have a handle, which the baby holds, and an insert, which contains the food. A two-pronged handle will be easiest for most babies to grasp at first, though they may graduate to a single handle later. Of the single-handled varieties, those with a squarer shape are generally easier to hold. The insert consists of either a molded silicone bulb, shaped like a giant pacifier with multiple small holes, or a flexible plastic net. As the baby chews on the bulb or net, the food is forced out of the holes. The advantage of a net is that it can accommodate large, irregularly shaped chunks of food, such as a piece of chicken or steak. Twisting the net to contain the piece of food tightly will discourage the baby from simply sucking on it and enable the food to be positioned on the part of the gum where the first molar will later erupt, so she can practice an up-and-down biting action and lateral tongue movements (see Rose, photo 65).

For most babies, a silicone insert will be more useful than a net. Silicone inserts come in different sizes. The ideal insert is one that is big enough to encourage an open jaw action but not so large that it makes graded chewing movements difficult. However, it's often a good idea to start with a smaller size, since this will be easier to place at the side of the mouth. A smaller insert also holds smaller amounts, so the baby is less likely to be overwhelmed if she happens to bite down hard. When she becomes proficient at using the feeder, a larger insert that can hold more food may be considered.

The amount of food that fits inside a small feeder insert is usually around one tablespoon. Initially, it's important to completely fill the feeder and to use foods that will pass through the holes easily, so that the baby is quickly rewarded for making the desired chewing movements. As the baby's chewing skills improve, the caregiver can be encouraged to introduce soft solid mashes that require greater jaw strength. Soon, the baby will be ready for foods such as raspberries—and eventually pieces of chicken or ground meat—that need more chewing to break them down sufficiently to pass through the holes. Extra care needs to be taken when selecting foods for babies who are at risk for aspiration; foods that release a thin liquid—orange segments, for example—are best avoided.

When using a silicone feeder, it's important to place the insert on top of the baby's lower gum, at the point where the first molar will appear. The idea is to encourage hand-to-mouth movements and chewing, not for the baby to suck on the insert in the center of her mouth. If hand-to-mouth facilitation is necessary, the caregiver should hold the baby's wrist gently with one hand and part of the handle of the feeder with the other. Eating is likely to be quite messy at first, especially with a thin puree. However, as the baby becomes proficient with the device, she will remove the food more cleanly and be ready for a refill more quickly. It can be helpful to have multiple feeders cued up, so she doesn't get frustrated waiting for the next mouthful of food.

Popsicles and frozen straws

In addition to starter strips, pre-loaded spoons, and silicone feeders, food popsicles and frozen straws are a useful way to help babies such as Luke (see page 26) work on their hand-to-mouth and chewing skills. They can also be handy for soothing the gums of babies who are teething. A popsicle made from human milk or infant formula is a great way to start, as the taste is already familiar. However, it's important to be aware that babies who have a history of aspiration may not be able to manage popsicles that melt into a thin liquid.

Babies need their popsicles to be short, so they are not unwieldy to lift, and fairly narrow, so they fit within their lips. Niko's popsicle (photo 25) is plenty big enough; mini popsicle molds are perfect. It's possible to make popsicles using a variety of ingredients, including calorie-rich foods (if there are growth concerns) and vegetables or fruit that can help with constipation. See Resources (page 259) for some useful recipe websites.

Frozen food straws (as used by Ethan, photo 26) are made using the type of reusable silicone straws originally designed for thick liquids, such as smoothies and milk shakes. The straw is cut in half (to make it easier for the baby to handle), filled with a soft, smooth food puree using a food pouch or syringe, and then frozen. As the baby holds one end of the straw and bites down on the other end, the puree will thaw and then dribble out, rewarding her efforts. Frozen straws enable practice at sustained chewing, resistive biting and pulling, and, when placed at the side of the mouth, lateral tongue movement.

Some babies don't like the coldness of food popsicles and straws, and those who are especially sensitive to temperature may reject them outright. Some parents find that straws are better tolerated than popsicles because the food is not in direct contact with the lips or the inside of the mouth; others report that popsicles work better because the handle itself is not cold.

Open-cup and straw drinking

Open-cup and straw drinking are especially important skills for babies with low muscle tone, or structural anomalies of the oral cavity. Both techniques use muscles of the lips, cheeks, and tongue that will be useful for speech as well as for eating; they are therefore a key part of ABLW.

Open-cup drinking

Open-cup drinking is a complex skill, requiring jaw stability as well as retraction (pulling back) and cupping of the tongue. Babies as young as 6 months can begin to drink from an open cup, although they will need some assistance at first. Small sips of liquid at the end of the meal, once the baby has lost interest in the food, is a good way to start. While some babies will be able to manage effectively from the outset, others will benefit from preparatory oral motor exercises, to help them avoid compensatory strategies (such as extending the tongue under the rim of the cup or biting on it). These actions, coupled with the overly wide jaw movements that most babies adopt in the early days, can result in a lot of liquid escaping, so a waterproof bib is a good idea. Full competence may not be achieved until two years of age, but with repeated practice, the baby will learn to keep her tongue inside her mouth, gain greater jaw stability, and use a more mature sucking action, making drinking progressively more effective and less messy.

The size of the cup is important. The diameter and curve of the rim should be proportionate to the size of the baby's mouth, to reduce the likelihood of loss of liquid at the corners of the mouth. A good first cup is a cut-out cup (see Thiago, photo 60). The cut-away rim allows the cup to be tipped without it touching the baby's nose (meaning she doesn't have to tilt her head back in order to drink) and enables the caregiver to see and control the flow of liquid. Babies who are more adept may be able to manage a small clear shot glass or medicine cup, or a commercially produced cup of similar size (see Resources, page 259). In general, the cup should be small and light enough for the baby to hold and tip easily, although babies with low muscle tone may manage better with a weighted cup, which will provide better feedback to guide their movements.

The choice of liquid for open-cup drinking is important because how it behaves makes a big difference to a baby's ability to manage the process safely and enjoyably (see page 000). Many babies will find thickened liquids or thinned purees, such as applesauce mixed with a little human milk, easier to manage at first. Initially, the cup will usually be held, or at least guided, by the caregiver, giving an extra degree of control. This will allow a fairly rapid transition to thinner liquids. However, when the baby starts to work on independent open-cup drinking, returning to a slightly thickened, nectar-like consistency (IDDSI level 2[3]) will help prevent her from being taken by surprise and reduce the likelihood of aspiration. While she is learning how to control the flow of liquid, the cup should be filled at least half full, so that she isn't required to tilt her head back in order to drink. This will provide additional protection for her airway.

Straw drinking

From around 7 to 9 months, straw drinking is also possible. This uses a different technique from that required for cup drinking, involving isolated lip movements and stronger activation of the cheek muscles (as demonstrated clearly by Emmett in photo 63), as well as tongue retraction and jaw stability. These skills may need to be worked on individually, as part of a pre-feeding program before the straw is introduced, with the aim of avoiding the baby's compensating for a lack of skill by using her tongue in a suckling movement or biting on the straw. Straw cups are easier for both babies and their care-givers to manage than attempting to hold a loose straw steady in an open cup. However, they tend to be bigger and heavier than open cups, so most babies will find a two-handled design easiest to manage, at least initially.

One way to introduce a baby to straw drinking is with a therapeutic squeezable straw cup, designed so that when the cup is gently compressed, the liquid is pushed up to the tip of the straw, allowing the caregiver to control the amount and the flow. This technique is known as facilitated straw drinking and it means the baby is rewarded for her sucking efforts while she figures out how to draw the liquid up for herself. Micah learned to drink from a straw using a cup like this (see Micah's story, page 211). An alternative is a straw cup with a valve that keeps the liquid at the top of the straw, making it easier for the baby to control. Once she has learned to draw the liquid up the straw independently and no longer needs the flow of liquid to be controlled for her, switching to a cup with a shorter straw will limit the amount that comes out at one time. The caregiver can also help the baby pace her sucking and avoid overfilling her mouth by voicing a one-two-three count. If she has difficulty swallowing, a thicker, more viscous liquid may be needed, although anything too thick will be almost impossible to draw up through the straw, tiring her and leaving her frustrated. If in doubt, the caregiver should check the flow themselves before offering the straw to the baby.

A third way to help a baby understand how a straw works is to use a straw as a pipette. This involves dipping a short straw (about 4 inches in length) into a glass of water, milk or thinned puree, then placing a finger on the opposite end, to hold the liquid in the straw. The open end of the straw is then offered to the baby's lips and—once she has given permission—gently inserted between them. When her lips are pursed around the tip of the straw, the finger is released briefly to allow a small amount of liquid to trickle into her mouth. Once she has dealt with that amount, some more can be allowed out of the straw. Starting with very small amounts and gradually increasing to larger volumes helps the baby to learn graded control.

It's possible to buy a series of therapeutic straws that promote jaw-lip-tongue dissociation.[4] Each of the different straws requires a slightly more advanced technique than the previous one, enabling the baby to work on oral motor skills like tongue retraction, lip rounding, and controlled, refined tongue movements. Being able to see their baby progressing through the stages can be very encouraging for parents, especially when progress is slow.

Therapeutic techniques

There are many therapeutic techniques used by therapists, three of which are a particularly good fit with ABLW. The "Sequential Oral Sensory Approach" created by psychologist Dr. Kay Toomey is designed for babies and children who have sensory issues that make it difficult for them to tolerate individual foods, colors, or textures.[5] It uses a hierarchy of typical developmental feeding skills, starting wherever the baby or child is most comfortable. For example, step one might be supporting the baby to tolerate food on her tray, the next step might be her picking the food up, and the third step an agreement to sniff the food—with the eventual goal that she will voluntarily eat some of it. The therapist or caregiver will slowly work their way up the hierarchy according to the baby's comfort level, sometimes taking a step backward if she has a setback. It's quite possible that the baby will be at different levels of the hierarchy with different foods; for example, being willing to eat broccoli but barely able to tolerate peas on her high chair tray, so it's important that the plan is designed around each baby individually.

Another useful technique is "food chaining," developed by speech pathologist Cheri Fraker.[6] In this method, chains, or links, are created from one food to another with the aim of expanding the baby's food repertoire. The first food in the chain will be something the baby already likes; the second food will be similar to the first but differ slightly in one or more characteristics, such as shape, size, or color. For example, if she is happy to eat mozzarella cheese slices, the chain may be to cheddar cheese slices. For a baby who enjoys raspberries, the chain may be to strawberries.

As well as her Get Permission Approach (see page 185), occupational therapist Marsha Dunn Klein has developed a variety of other responsive feeding techniques. In "around the bowl," the therapist puts two foods into opposite sides of a bowl— one that the baby likes, and another that is new to her or that she likes less. The therapist begins by offering the preferred food, then the less-liked food, noting the baby's reaction. If she reacts negatively, the therapist goes "around the bowl" and returns to the preferred food, slowly stretching the baby to incorporate a new food or texture, without pressure. Both "food chaining" and "around the bowl" were used effectively with Micah (see page 211).

Tailoring the feeding plan to the baby

The age at which solid foods are introduced, and the speed with which an individual baby is able to feed herself without help, will depend on many different factors, such as the degree of prematurity or developmental delay (if any), the nature and timing of surgeries, and the ability and enthusiasm of her parents to follow through with the necessary exercises. A baby with a feeding aversion will require a very different approach from either a baby with neurological impairment or a baby with a cleft palate. Each will need an individualized plan based on the nature of her condition, her medical history and prognosis, and her family situation. Similarly, the feeding plan appropriate for one baby may be quite unlike the plan for a baby with a different skill set, even if their history and circumstances are similar.

Common to all feeding plans is not to pressure the baby to eat particular foods or specified amounts. This will not be easy for parents who are concerned about their baby's weight or who have their own deep-seated issues over food. They may try to extend mealtimes, perhaps by playing games; they may coerce the baby to eat; or they may want to take over the feeding with a spoon or pouch at the end of the meal, just to satisfy themselves that she has eaten enough. It can be hard to accept that these behaviors are counterproductive and will usually make the baby less likely to eat willingly.

Babies with a history of aversion and/or sensory issues

Babies who are feeding averse, or who have heightened sensory responses to food, can easily feel overwhelmed or under pressure to eat. For those whose development is otherwise typical, a regular BLW hands-off approach, beginning with sticks or strips of vegetables, fruit, and meat, is ideal. Care should be taken to avoid putting too much food in front of the baby at one time or encouraging her to "Take a bite," since both of these things can feel threatening. If she is wary of the high chair, she may feel safer sitting on her mom or dad's lap until her confidence grows. Pre-loaded spoons and/or silicone feeders may be useful initially, since they will provide some distance between the baby's hands and the food and make it more likely that she will bring the food to her mouth. It may take her many weeks to become confident to feed herself, but the key is for her to be in full control of her eating at all times.

Feeding aversion can be incredibly frustrating for parents because the reasons for the behavior are not always obvious. They, too, will benefit from the support of a knowledgeable feeding therapist. There may be frequent setbacks, such as when the baby is teething or sick or has a skin reaction to a food she has eaten. With patience, gentle encouragement, and positive reinforcement, she will gradually desensitize to the unfamiliar sensations. Her progression to accepting solid foods may take a bit longer than for her peers, but a responsive, baby-led approach will help overcome the challenges and foster a positive relationship with food.

As a mother of preemie twins who suffered from reflux and bottle aversion, I quickly learned that starting solids through BLW would have immense benefits. Self-feeding and exploring food restored their enjoyment of eating. All babies benefit from being able to self-feed on their own terms.

Christiana Scott, mother of Andrew and Wyatt and
founder of Real Food Littles

Babies with neurodevelopmental issues

Babies whose neurodevelopment is impaired, for example, those with Down syndrome or Prader-Willi syndrome, commonly struggle with eye-hand coordination and hand-to-mouth movements. They can find it especially difficult to coordinate their hands together to hold a large piece of food and guide it to their mouth and may favor one hand over the other. They may struggle to lower their gaze, in which case placing food on the high chair tray for them to pick up, and perhaps tapping gently on the tray to draw their attention to it, will be an important element of the feeding plan. Many babies with these challenges find large foods easier to manage if they first lean toward the food with their mouth and then have their hands guided to make contact with it, either one at a time or together. Some will be able to use one hand in this way before they can use both simultaneously, so they will need the food to be supported for them from underneath.

In addition to issues of coordination and dexterity, babies with atypical neurodevelopment may have weak jaw muscles. They may therefore need extra support and practice to develop the necessary skills before self-feeding becomes possible. However, there is no reason why, in parallel with a pre-feeding program, some of this additional practice can't be done with actual food, using therapeutic feeding techniques such as facilitation (see page 188), provided that the shape, size, and texture of the foods are carefully chosen. This will be more interesting and rewarding for the baby than a plastic toy or teether and will make the transition to self-feeding easier.

> Evan is my second child, but with his diagnosis of Down syndrome I didn't know what to expect with feeding. I was very pleasantly surprised by how quickly he started transitioning to solids, and it was a bonus that we could work toward speech and occupational therapy goals with food!
>
> Carolyn, mother of Evan, who has Down syndrome

Food placement: a way to promote chewing and jaw strength

An exercise that can help to strengthen the force a baby can apply with her jaw, while also stimulating tongue lateralization and a munching pattern, is food placement. This can be done using either a fork (known as therapeutic fork feeding[7]) or the tip of a finger, although the latter should not be attempted if the baby's molars have already come in (because of the risk of your being bitten!). The technique can be used briefly a few times during a meal in which the baby is otherwise self-feeding, alternating sides to encourage the even development of the muscles.

Version 1 (as used with Adiel; see page 149): The therapist or caregiver uses a small fork (preferably one with narrow, slightly curved tines, such as a cocktail fork or child's fork) to spear a small piece of a soft solid food. They then turn the fork so the tines curve downward and—having gained the baby's permission—use it to place the food on the lower first molar (or on the gum at the spot where the first molar will later erupt). The baby will usually bite down spontaneously, with the desired chewing movement. The fork is withdrawn slowly, as the baby closes her jaws on the food.

Version 2: The therapist or caregiver uses the soft pad of their finger to place the food on the gum. They then apply gentle downward pressure and wait for the baby to respond by pushing upward. As the baby starts to chew, the finger can be slowly withdrawn to allow her to carry on. If necessary, the caregiver can keep their finger inside the baby's cheek, resting against the outside of the gum, to help keep the food in place for repetitive chewing practice.

Initial food explorations may be very brief and difficult for the baby. However, with practice, she will become more purposeful in bringing strips of food to her mouth and her aim will improve, so that she no longer needs facilitation. For some babies this will happen very quickly (as with Sophia; see page 133) maybe after just one taste; others will require support for considerably longer. Often the feel of the food on the baby's gums (especially if she is teething) will motivate her to want to manage the process herself. Once she is doing well with bringing starter strips to her mouth independently, she may be ready to move seamlessly to finger foods and pursue a classic BLW path. Alternatively, she may need a further transition period using one or more bridge devices.

Babies with motor or structural challenges

Babies with motor difficulties or conditions affecting the anatomy and function of the mouth, throat, and/or the respiratory and gastrointestinal system will usually require an adapted version of BLW, particularly if chewing movements are compromised. Depending on the nature of their condition they may benefit initially from mouthing and chewing practice using starter food strips. However, to ensure adequate nutrition and sufficient intake of calories during this time, they may also need to be offered mashed or pureed textures using one or more bridge devices. This will allow the baby to enjoy exploring and tasting food while increasing jaw strength, improving chewing skills, ensuring safe swallowing, and enhancing her confidence with food. If she requires additional support to manipulate the spoon or feeder, the caregiver can provide gentle facilitation (see page 188), in much the same way as for a baby with neurodevelopmental difficulties.

Babies who have been tube fed

Babies who have been fed by tube for extended periods may have had little or no experience of food in their mouth. They are also unlikely to have had the opportunity to look at or touch food. A child-directed approach, in which the baby can pick and choose which foods she wants to eat while simultaneously honing her feeding skills and catching up on missed learning, is a hugely beneficial way to support her transition to eating by mouth.

Phasing out the tube should be guided by a feeding team, which may include physicians, dietitians, and feeding therapists, to ensure smooth progress. However, there should ideally be no rush to get rid of the tube, since its ongoing use means that there need be no concerns about weight gain, or pressure on the baby to consume large amounts of food by mouth. This will allow her the freedom to become acquainted with food at her own pace and to enjoy making new discoveries.

> As we had spoon fed all of our five other kids, I thought we would transition Faith to solids the same way. None of the others were self-feeding like Faith is now at such a young age, so I really didn't think this method would work. Now I think it is amazing how she transitioned from a tube—after having it for 10 months—to feeding herself. It's been great!
>
> Denise, mother of Faith, who has Down syndrome

Progression toward full self-feeding

Every baby is different, and the rate at which they move through the preparatory and transitional stages to independent self-feeding using their hands will vary according to their individual history, developmental skill level, and degree of motor strength. Some babies' oral skills will be ahead of their fine motor skills—and vice versa—meaning that progression through the various food textures may or may not mirror the baby's ability to get food to her mouth. The key is for parents and therapists to find a happy medium of challenging the baby just enough that she continues to work on the necessary skills, without making the task so difficult that she becomes frustrated.

While the start is often slow, once babies can grasp individual strips of food and take them to their mouth, they can progress rapidly in several directions at once. They can begin to hold and gnaw on large foods, feed themselves with meltable solids, pick up small pieces of food using a refined thumb-and-forefinger pincer grasp, take bites out of foods such as sandwiches, and eventually manage mixed textured foods. They will also be able to cope with having a range of shapes and textures presented together, which will help them become adept at applying different skills in the space of the same meal. The "Self-feeding ladder" shows what a typical progression through the stages of ABLW might look like.

Self-feeding ladder

The list below illustrates what an individual baby's progress through the various stages of ABLW might look like.
The exact order is variable, depending on each baby's needs and limitations, and some skills may be worked on simultaneously. All the steps will usually be accompanied by practice at drinking, first from an open cup and, later, via a straw.

- Starter strips, frozen straws, popsicles, feeders, and/or pre-loaded spoons, first with facilitation, then offered from caregiver's hand for baby to grasp and take to her mouth unaided, then placed on high chair tray for her to pick up with palmar grasp

- Introduction of pre-dipped or pre-loaded starter strips (e.g., celery dipped in hummus), with encouragement for baby to dip

- Use of food teethers to work on gnawing, chewing, and jaw strength
- Food mashes placed on high chair tray, to be raked and picked up with palmar grasp
- Large foods held or supported by caregiver, so baby can lean forward for tastes and begin to hold them herself
- Large foods placed on high chair tray, for baby to grip with both hands and gnaw
- Practice at holding and taking graded bites from soft solid strips (e.g., banana or avocado) with caregiver initially assisting and grading bite size with their finger (as illustrated by Owen in photo 66)
- Practice in graded gnawing on meltable solid strips, moving to clean bites through the strip and eventually eating small meltable solid pieces
- Practice with resistive food strips, for biting and pulling
- Small pieces of soft solids and/or meltable solids, offered first from caregiver's palm halfway between tray and baby's mouth, gradually moving caregiver's palm downward to touch the tray, so baby has to look and reach down to get them
- Small pieces of soft solids and/or meltable solids offered between caregiver's index finger and thumb, to help facilitate a pincer grasp
- Small pieces of soft solids, placed on high chair tray (may be rolled in a dry food to reduce slipperiness)
- Small pieces of soft solids, offered on a pre-loaded fork
- Self-feeding of mixed textures and composite foods
- Small pieces of food that require more chewing
- Firmer food strips (for eating rather than as starter strips or teethers)
- Independent use of spoon and/or fork

Practicing feeding skills does not have to be restricted to mealtimes: While the baby, her parents, and her therapist are working on one skill, using therapeutic feeding techniques and practicing with real food, the therapist may be setting up the next and more challenging feeding step using oral motor exercises and nonfood therapeutic devices as part of a pre-feeding program (see page 126). For example, a baby who is using a pre-loaded spoon with mashes may be introduced to a silicone teether to encourage repetitive up and down chewing movements prior to transitioning to a silicone feeder or to finger foods. By working together on several areas in parallel, the parent and therapist will enable the baby to make as rapid progress as possible in all aspects of eating, thereby accelerating her path to full self-feeding.

> We have seen incredible success with a baby-led weaning approach with decreasing oral aversion, weaning off feeding tubes, building oral skills, and creating positive mealtime experiences, even for babies who are considered at risk for feeding difficulties.
>
> Kary Rappaport, and Kimberly Grenawitzke, pediatric occupational therapists

MICAH'S STORY

Jill's account

MICAH'S HISTORY

Micah is his parents' fourth child. He was born with a congenital diaphragmatic hernia (CDH), which meant that his abdominal organs protruded into his chest cavity, making breathing difficult. At 2 days old he underwent a surgical repair of the hernia. He spent six weeks in the neonatal intensive care unit (NICU) and was prescribed medication for reflux. I first met Micah's mom in my role as lactation consultant, and we discussed how she could protect her milk supply with pumping until he would be allowed home. At the time I had no idea that ten months later I would be their feeding therapist.

Micah was discharged home at 6 weeks. At that stage he was being fed his mom's milk, mostly by bottle and sometimes via a nasogastric tube. His mom had breastfed her three older children and worked hard to establish breastfeeding with Micah, finally achieving it when he was 3 months old. Micah's parents began introducing purees when he reached 4 months and started offering him table finger foods from 7 months. This was not a great success and, at 11 months, his physical therapist referred him to me. At this stage he was being spoon fed with rice, oatmeal, and mixed-grain cereals, as well as commercial Stage 2 vegetable and fruit purees. He was breast-feeding four times a day and receiving 4 to 6 ounces of his mom's milk by bottle, but he was struggling to gain weight.

MICAH'S FEEDING THERAPY INTERVENTION AND PROGRESS

At my initial evaluation I noted that Micah had an open-mouth resting posture, a sign of low muscle tone. During our session he also had what appeared to be a few reflux episodes, involving random coughing, and he appeared guarded about food. If he got any on his hands, he would visually examine them and seemed bothered by it. He readily accepted commercial Stage 2 carrots and cereal when his mom spoon fed him, but when given a spoon pre-loaded with the same foods, he would drop it on the floor. He refused mashed banana, then started to refuse the carrot puree, so it was clear we needed to tread lightly. He brought meltable snack foods to his mouth for tastes but he wouldn't do the same with a silicone feeder, and he turned away from both an open cup and a straw cup.

After the evaluation I recommended weekly feeding therapy sessions. An early priority was to help Micah with his posture, as he tended to slouch and would tire easily. Struggling to sit upright for extended periods of time limited how long he was able to stay focused on eating. His physical therapist helped to arrange optimal seating, including support for his feet, and we eventually found a high-backed booster seat. I encouraged his parents to create family meals and to have all the food on the table before putting Micah in his high chair. I also suggested that they have him in the kitchen with them during prepping and cooking, to help him become desensitized to the sights and smells of food. Meanwhile, the dietitian and I carried out joint therapy sessions with the family, to help ensure his ongoing weight gain and intake of necessary micronutrients.

I explained to Micah's parents the importance of seeking his permission before helping him with feeding, and we implemented an "around the bowl" technique (see page 200) to encourage him to accept new foods. We also began to work on self-feeding, using spoons pre-loaded with his preferred purees as well as

starter food strips such as steamed broccoli. We experimented
briefly with food popsicles and frozen bananas on a stick but
abandoned them because Micah disliked the cold temperature.

Micah really liked crunchy meltable snack foods. To help
increase his calorie intake we dipped them in cream cheese
and peanut butter, and we also created little sandwich crackers
with these as fillings. We began introducing other liquids once
he turned 1, starting with coconut water and gradually adding
coconut milk until he was drinking straight coconut milk. Then
we did the same thing to help him transition from coconut milk
to cow's milk. At around 14 months, the dietitian suggested that
Micah's parents add cream to his cereal and oils to his purees to
ensure they were calorie-rich. She also advised them to fortify his
cow's milk drinks with powdered toddler formula.

Another successful idea was to present small pieces of cereal in
a mound of peanut butter on Micah's tray, then tell him they were
"stuck" and have him pull them out. He liked toast strips, though
we had to cue him to "bite and pull" them or he would stuff
the whole strip in his mouth. But he made it clear—by throwing
them—that he wouldn't tolerate "wet" foods such as raspberries.
We played a game in which he would feed his mom foods he
didn't like, to get him to touch them without feeling pressured.
Gradually, he started to accept slices of cheese and to dip his
finger in nut butter and transfer it to his mouth. We also used food
chaining (see page 200), offering Micah a food that he liked: for
example, peanut butter, followed by a similarly textured food with
a slightly different taste, like almond butter.

When Micah first began wanting to eat table foods, he didn't
have the skills to chew them thoroughly, and we had to be careful
to avoid choking, as he was inclined to overstuff his mouth.
We therefore did some therapeutic feeding work, placing soft,

solid strips and meltable solids on his gums, working through
Overland and Merkel-Walsh's chewing hierarchy (see page 128)
and encouraging him to use repetitive, graded biting movements
and take clean and complete bites. Beginning at 11 months, we
focused on straw drinking as an alternative to the breast and
bottle, using a therapeutic straw cup. Micah began to enjoy
a coconut water and coconut milk mixture offered this way.
However, he struggled to drink independently, so we worked on
activating his cheek muscles and stimulating lip rounding. He was
so proud of himself when, at the age of 18 months, he eventually
mastered it!

At around 13 months, Micah began refusing to breast-feed
when he was awake, nursing only at night or first thing in the
morning, when he was sleepy. He also started rejecting the bottle,
so his mom had to rely on overnight and sleepy feeds to keep him
hydrated. At 15 months he started occupational therapy consisting
of exercises and activities to improve his core strength and to
create a calm environment, to help him stay focused and relaxed
through activities that were hard for him.

At 17 months, after six months of feeding therapy and having
recently stopped his reflux medication, Micah began to refuse
purees. However, he was feeding himself effectively with a variety
of snack foods. He also liked strips of toast, cheese, and waffle.
As his molars started to appear, his chewing skills improved
markedly, and from around 18 months it became less of a struggle
for his parents to maintain his calorie and nutrient intake. From
24 months of age, he was able to move on to more typical table
foods such as cheese slices and cucumber.

At nearly 3 years old Micah now eats a wide variety of table
foods and can even manage a whole peeled apple. He enjoys
breaded fish, chicken nuggets, and bacon. He self-feeds all his

meals and drinks from a straw cup. He tends to eat quickly, but he chews effectively and swallows safely. He is still tentative and guarded around foods that are not his favorites, but he is generally willing to try new foods and to assimilate them slowly into his diet. He plays a full part in family mealtimes and truly enjoys them.

DISCUSSION

Progress with self-feeding and more textured foods was slow, owing to Micah's anxiety around eating. This appeared to stem from initial respiratory problems caused by the hernia, and interventions like placement of the nasogastric tube. He would also have setbacks when he would get sick or was teething. From very early on he would push away unfamiliar foods, say "all done," and want to get down from his chair.

The family did a great job of respecting Micah's cues. Even his siblings understood what was needed and never pushed him to eat something, instead allowing it to be his choice. His mom found a neat way to get him to try new foods, which was to offer the food to his siblings first, saying, for example, "Who wants pizza?" Micah wound up trying many different foods this way. He still has the occasional setback but he is resilient enough to recover quickly. The ABLW approach has undoubtedly helped him transition into a safe and happy eater.

Micah's mom's perspective

We were initially fairly confident about introducing solid foods to Micah. Not having experienced any major feeding issues with our older three children, we expected to introduce solids as we always had and for the outcome to be as it always was. However, like all things with Micah's development, nothing went quite as we expected.

Micah is unique, with every milestone hard-fought and achieved in a new and different way than it was with our other children. In hindsight I'm not sure why I expected his feeding journey to be smooth. After all, we brought him home from the hospital at 6 weeks old on a nasogastric feeding tube to supplement his breast- and bottle feeding. Even though he had the tube for only about two more weeks, his feeding journey was still a challenging one. We had to work hard to get enough volume and weight gain when he switched to oral-only feeding.

Solid feeding went fairly well for the first few months of baby grain cereals and pureed vegetables and fruits. It wasn't until we started with table food that we became concerned. Many meals and weeks passed, and still he would not accept one bite of anything that wasn't a spoon-fed cereal or puree. We were encouraged by Micah's pediatrician and physical therapist to simply give him time, and we were reassured that he would probably come around. However, weeks turned into months, and we found ourselves at a loss as to what to do.

After several months of our unsuccessful attempts at introducing solid table food, Micah began refusing his purees and cereals. He was not gaining weight, and most concerningly, he stopped taking in liquids, refusing both breast and bottle. Jill fit us into her schedule right away and introduced a whole new approach to feeding Micah. It took a lot of time and patience, but by completely flipping from the mindset of "feeding Micah" to "Micah feeding himself," we slowly began to see results. Once we started offering him his cereals and purees on a pre-loaded spoon, instead of spooning them into his mouth, I could see him becoming more relaxed. I had to understand that, from Micah's perspective, new things going in his mouth were scary to him. He'd been intubated for ten days after birth, with other medical interventions over the following weeks. He was cautious, and solid food was a new concept. But, by changing our approach and giving him all the control, we began to see results.

Once Micah became familiar with self-feeding from pre-loaded spoons, we again began offering some solid table food. Jill taught us how to model eating it ourselves and make it a no-pressure situation. She also showed us how bigger food is better than smaller, giving Micah better control of his bite and how much to put in his mouth. All this made him feel safer and calmer. Still, we had two entire months of offering him food, him exploring it, and it ending up on the floor. Inside, I was so frustrated and nervous that my child would never eat real food, but on the outside I was completely calm, drawing no attention to the food that was all over my floor and not in my child's stomach.

Then one day, when I was barely looking, Micah worked up the courage to take the smallest bite of a teething biscuit. Then he took another bite, and another. What a breakthrough! This was the beginning. We still had a long road ahead of us, but when Micah took those first few bites at 13 months old, I cried. His self-feeding journey was all on his own timeline. Did he trust the food? Did he trust us? Well, now, almost two years later Micah does completely trust us—and the food we give him. If something is new, he knows that we are never going to make him eat it, so it's no problem for it to sit next to him on the table. He is in control.

Micah still has a way to go but he is happy and healthy, gaining weight and progressing in all areas of his development. I certainly couldn't ask for more.

MICAH'S DAD'S PERSPECTIVE

When we began feeding therapy for Micah, I was apprehensive and nervous. Our littlest boy, unlike our three older children who transitioned easily to solid foods, was not thriving and not gaining weight. I feared that he was spiraling downward. As breast-feeding was increasingly unable to meet his needs and his purees and cereals were slipping, I felt helpless. So when Jill suggested, "Let Micah decide. Just model and offer new foods, without actually directly feeding him, and with absolutely no pressure," it was very hard to trust and be patient. It felt unnatural compared to the parent-led mealtime routines we had established and practiced in our home for ten years.

I was grateful for Jill's explanations about how Micah's oral aversion was likely linked to all the negative experiences he had in the NICU; it helped me understand that forcing the issue would be counterproductive and undermine his trust of food and, ultimately, of us as his parents. Progress was incremental at first— but steady—and gradually picked up momentum. It was, at times, frustrating for us to prepare a variety of foods and then see hardly any of it make it into Micah's mouth—and less still into his belly. However, just as his trust in our mealtime routines and confidence to explore food grew, so did my own trust in the process and my motivation to stick with it for Micah's sake. Now, as he wolfs down his meals, heavily loaded with his preferred items but (mostly) hitting all of the food groups, I feel deep relief, satisfaction, and gratitude. We still sometimes just stop and watch him eat and can't help but smile, thinking about how far he's come!

9
.....

Common Parental Concerns

The prospect of your child handling pieces of food and feeding himself while he's still a baby can feel daunting, even when you know how many benefits it will have for him. You may encounter questions and criticism from family and friends—and even some health professionals. Your baby may react in ways that alarm or puzzle you or seem not to make any progress. This chapter explores some of these common concerns and suggests how to overcome them so you can support your baby in his exciting journey to independent eating.

Engaging support

Although baby-led weaning isn't a new idea, in recent times it hasn't been the accepted way to introduce babies to solid food. Most parents, grandparents, and professionals in the developed world are only just discovering it. The first reaction of many is to distrust what isn't familiar to them, especially when they don't yet see it reflected in mainstream guidance. They worry that it will harm babies or expose them to risk. Spoon feeding is seen as safer, even though it has been around for far shorter a time and has little or no research to support it. Sharing this book with the skeptics in your life may help them understand how ABLW works.

Most people who are skeptical, either about BLW in general or about adapting it for a baby who has feeding challenges, find themselves won over when they see it in practice. It's hard to be critical, faced with a baby who is clearly enjoying engaging with food. They may be alarmed, initially, when they see your baby gagging until they understand that this is a normal reflex that may even help him learn to eat safely. It can be helpful to remind older family members and friends that they, too, probably had some child-rearing ideas that their parents disapproved of; knowledge increases with each generation, and you, like them, are doing the best you can with the information that's available.

> When I first heard Ethan had Down syndrome, I didn't know what to expect. When he began eating solid food, my son and his wife explained they would not be using a spoon. I was puzzled, skeptical, and worried he would not get the nutrition he needed. I watched Ethan using his own hands to pick up pieces of avocado or mashed hard-boiled eggs with mayonnaise and get them to his mouth. It was messy, yet he was successfully feeding himself.
>
> Jill, grandmother/grandma of Ethan, 15 months

Finding the right team of professionals to support you and getting started early in your baby's life can be crucial, especially in situations where you know that it is inevitable that he will face delays and challenges. Not all therapists have the same experience and knowledge, and your baby's journey will be easier if as many of his doctors and therapists as possible (and especially the lead feeding therapist) are supportive of the ABLW approach and have some understanding of the rationale behind it. Planning ahead (see chapter 5) will enable your child to establish a strong gross motor foundation and develop pre-feeding skills, which in turn will translate to an easier transition to solids. It may also prevent or minimize more difficult and complicated feeding problems once actual food is offered.

You may find it helpful to identify sources of support from other parents who are doing BLW, and from professionals who actively support and promote it. There are currently many websites, apps, and social media groups devoted to the approach, including some that are specific to babies whose development is atypical. See page 259 for just some of the resources you can tap into. Be cautious, though, of following recommendations you may see on social media accounts and make sure that the person you choose to follow is a legitimate health care professional, rather than someone basing their advice on their own personal experiences. However good their ideas may seem, their baby is not your baby. If you and he are encountering feeding challenges, it is safest to adhere to information from an experienced professional.

I didn't give too much thought to feeding solids until we had an event in the NICU where Viviana choked while feeding on a bottle. Because of this, I became nervous for what could be ahead with the twins' feeding journey. I also think that being exposed to so much on the internet, while it can be helpful, can also make you question what you are/aren't doing, especially with feeding, when you see babies doing more than yours.

Brie, mother of Liliana and Viviana,
born at 28 weeks' gestation

Trying to implement ABLW without professional support is likely to be stressful and may be unsafe. If your baby's therapist and health care providers are not supportive of ABLW, you may wish to seek out other feeding and medical professionals whose thinking is more in line with your parenting and feeding philosophies. Other families who have successfully done ABLW or BLW may be able to recommend someone in your area that they have worked with and who is supportive and knowledgeable. Alternatively, it may be possible to make contact with a professional who supports ABLW and who would offer online or phone consultations. If it is not feasible for you to change providers, you may be able to educate those you do consult by showing them videos of your child, or of other children following ABLW—for example, on professionally supported social media accounts—to help demonstrate the effectiveness of the approach. You could also point them to literature and research papers about BLW, many of which can be found in the Notes section of this book.

Managing Milk Feeds

Milk feedings are likely to continue to be an important source of nourishment for your baby until he is at least one year, and possibly older. Human milk or infant formula is more nutrient-dense than any other single food, so it's important not to dampen his appetite for it. He will discover gradually that solid food can fill his belly but, until this happens (probably not before he's 9 months old, at the earliest), it may be frustrating for him to be offered solid food when he's hungry and looking forward to a milk feed. The best approach is to offer the breast or bottle shortly before a shared mealtime is planned, so that he is happy and ready for a new experience. Soon after his eating becomes more purposeful you will notice him taking less at his milk feeds, or perhaps skipping one of them altogether. Following his lead as to how quickly he cuts down his milk intake will help ensure that the weaning process happens at a pace that works for him.

Potential responses to solid foods

There are some behaviors that occur frequently when babies feed themselves, for example, throwing food, using the tongue to push it out or "pocketing" it in the cheeks, overstuffing the mouth, gagging, and coughing. These responses are especially common in babies who have difficulty with chewing, who have sensory issues or a feeding aversion, or who are otherwise fearful or anxious about eating.

Throwing food

There are many reasons why, when babies are feeding themselves, food ends up on the floor. A baby of 6 or 7 months will
commonly sweep food off his high chair tray with his arm or
lose the piece he was holding when his hand opens reflexively
while his attention is elsewhere. This is entirely unintentional
and the baby will often not be aware that it has happened. A
month or two later he will notice food falling, and soon after
that he'll realize that he can make this happen. This typically
leads to experiments involving purposeful throwing or dropping of food, in order to see or hear it fall to the floor. It's an
exciting science lesson!

From around 8 months, babies sometimes throw pieces of
food because they see something more appealing that they
would like to eat instead. Alternatively, they may do it for a
reaction from their caregiver, or it may be a way for them to
communicate that they are done eating. Pushing food off the
tray can also be a sign of frustration, for example, if the baby
is struggling to pick up a very slippery food. Babies with a
feeding aversion may throw food to avoid eating, or because
of a heightened sensory response to a less-well-liked food, or
one that they don't regularly eat.

To respond appropriately, it's essential to try to understand
why your baby is throwing food. If it happens after a period of
contented exploration or eating, then it's likely a sign that he
is bored or no longer hungry. In that case the best response is
first to offer a different food and then, if that doesn't work, to
end the meal. If it's being done to gain your attention, ignoring
the behavior itself, and instead redirecting his attention (for

example, by smiling and talking, or by offering a drink), will tend to encourage him to find other ways to communicate his needs. Another option is to provide a "No, thank you" bowl into which, with demonstrations and gentle reminders from you, he can learn to put food he doesn't want, instead of throwing it on the floor. Addie's parents used this technique to help when Addie began throwing food (see Addie's story, page 113).

Ejecting and pocketing food

Using the tongue to push food out of the mouth can be simply the normal, healthy reaction of a baby who has taken a bite that is too big for him to chew. It's a way for him to protect himself him from choking, and it allows him to study the food and perhaps tackle it differently when he puts it back into his mouth. Alternatively, ejecting food can be a sign that the baby is struggling to chew, because his sensory feedback or skill level is not up to the task. It can also be a way of avoiding swallowing food, perhaps because of a sensory aversion or history of reflux or choking, or a food allergy.

Pocketing food in the cheeks (like a chipmunk) is another way for a baby to avoid swallowing food. This, too, may be a sensory-based issue involving specific textures, or be related to a history of reflux or choking, or of being force-fed. It can also be the result of an inability to break the food down sufficiently to allow it to be swallowed easily and safely. Occasionally, small amounts of food get pocketed unintentionally, when they become caught in between the gum and the cheek or lodged in the roof of the mouth, especially if the baby lacks the refined movements of the tongue necessary to extract them. If you think your baby may have pocketed some food, a quick check inside his mouth at the end of the meal (with his permission) is a useful precaution.

If your baby continues to push out or pocket partially chewed food, the answer may be to go back—either to foods that require less chewing, to foods he finds easier to manage, or to smaller amounts that can be chewed and swallowed successfully. You may like to try offering him occasional sips of a drink to encourage him to swallow more frequently. However, it's important to avoid insisting that he drink in an effort to "wash down" the food. Indeed, you should always make sure he doesn't have any food pieces in his mouth before offering liquid; if a baby is unable to chew a bite effectively, and is avoiding swallowing in order to protect himself, pushing sips (or mouthfuls) of liquid will not be helpful and could lead to choking or aspiration.

If your baby's therapist has devised a pre-feeding program for him, they may wish to adapt it to enable him to work on more advanced chewing skills in between meals, perhaps using a silicone teether to build jaw strength and tongue movement. This can be done alongside therapeutic feeding exercises aimed at tackling foods that are more difficult to chew, such as offering pieces of chicken inside a netted feeder.

Overstuffing

When babies first begin to handle strips of food, they commonly try to stuff the whole piece into their mouth or take too big a bite. This is a normal part of learning and isn't true overstuffing. They just need to be encouraged to spit the piece out and try again. If, after a few attempts your baby is struggling to figure out how much to bite off, you can help him by holding the strip with your index finger and thumb just beyond where you want his gums or teeth to meet, then wait for him to give you permission to place the exposed part in his mouth so he can bite it (as Owen's parent is doing in photo 66). For an older baby or toddler, who is able to understand simple imagery, Marsha Dunn Klein's "bite size discretion" technique may be helpful.[1] This involves inviting the child to take bites of varying sizes, such as "a mouse bite" or "an elephant bite," using pictures and gestures to illustrate the difference.

Some babies bite off a small amount but then keep taking more bites without having swallowed the first one. This type of overstuffing can be a sign that the baby lacks the necessary skills to chew the food effectively (see Luan's story, page 178). It's common in babies with low muscle tone and reduced oral sensory feedback, who don't realize there is too much in their mouth until it's too late. It is also frequently seen in babies who have been given all their food as purees, and who have therefore not learned that some foods require chewing before they can be swallowed. If your baby is struggling to deal with a large mouthful, try inviting him to eject it and start again. Encouragement to chew and swallow after each bite will help him discover how to prevent the problem from recurring.

Gagging and coughing

Gagging and coughing are normal, healthy reflexes that are often triggered when babies are learning to eat (see "Protective mechanisms related to eating," page 70). Provided the baby is sitting in an upright position, these reflexes will usually operate effectively. However, to minimize the risk of choking, some extra precautions may need to be taken for babies with challenging conditions.

Some babies are more prone to gagging than others. Those with sensory-based feeding issues, and those who have had negative experiences related to oral feedings (perhaps due to a complicated medical history or having been pressured to eat), may have a more pronounced and exaggerated gag reflex that persists for a longer period of time than it does for their typical peers. Babies who have difficulty making upward and sideways movements of their tongue, such as those with a neuromotor disorder or a tongue-tie, may also gag more easily than other babies; if a piece of food gets stuck on the middle of their tongue, their attempts to move it to the side for chewing can easily trigger a gag response. In these situations, it is important to proceed slowly, increasing the texture and variety of the food very gradually to allow the baby plenty of time to adjust, while simultaneously working on the necessary feeding skills.

Babies with swallowing issues, such as weakness or lack of coordination of the laryngeal muscles or a tendency to aspirate, are at greater risk for choking, so it's essential that any liquids offered are of a safe consistency. If the baby is struggling to manage thin liquids, it's important to avoid solid foods that may turn into thin liquids, like a melting popsicle, or those that release a thin liquid when bitten into, such as orange segments. Other liquids can generally be thickened to make them safe before they are offered. Foods, such as cookies, that generate dry crumbs also present a risk for babies who have difficulty swallowing, so they may need to be avoided.

Some babies with neurodevelopmental challenges will have specific recommendations made for the appropriate consistency of food and liquid to be offered (see page 177). For example, foods may need to be pureed or soft and bite-size, and liquids anything from thin to moderately thick, until the baby is able to manage more challenging formats. In general, having your baby's feeding therapist guide you in the selection of food and drink for him will help the solid food transition go more smoothly.

A high-arched palate, commonly seen in some syndromes, or tethered oral tissues (such as a tongue-tie) can cause food to become impacted in the roof of the mouth while the baby is eating. This is especially likely if his chewing skills are underdeveloped or if he has limited oral sensory awareness. The problem is that everything can appear fine until the food gets dislodged: If it breaks free during the meal it may cause gagging or combine with the next bite to make a mouthful that is too big for him to manage; if it goes unnoticed and becomes detached later, when he is playing or sleeping, there is a risk that he could choke. If you know that food is likely to get stuck against your baby's palate (or pocketed in his cheeks), you can watch for him taking bites with no swallowing in between and then make a game of checking the inside of his mouth—especially at the end of the meal.

Optimal positioning is key to minimizing gagging and coughing incidents and keeping mealtimes safe and enjoyable for you and your baby. Selecting which foods he can safely self-feed, based on his chewing skill level, will also be protective. Clearly, foods whose shape or texture present a choking risk for all babies (such as pieces of nuts, small round fruits, and coin-shaped pieces of carrot or hot dog) should be strenuously avoided for babies who have any sort of feeding difficulties, but so too should foods such as crackers that snap readily or behave unpredictably, or that release crumbs that disperse all over the mouth. It's also risky to assume that all puff-type snacks are equally meltable—some require more chewing than others in order to break them down, and some can become quite difficult to chew if not consumed quickly after the bag is opened. It's a good idea to check any food you are not sure of yourself before offering it to your baby. A baby who doesn't have the ability to move food pieces from the center of his mouth to the side for chewing may need a longer period of practice with textured mashes, starter strips, and silicone feeders, as well as pre-feeding chewing exercises, before he can advance to taking bites from strips of food or managing more complex or mixed textures.

What if we're already spoon feeding?

It's not unusual for parents or their advisers to want to switch to ABLW after they have already started spoon feeding. This may be because they have only just heard about this approach, because a previous health professional did not promote it, because complementary feeding began before the baby was 6 months old, or because spoon feeding is not going well. The good news is that it's never too late to transition to a child-directed way of doing things.

A useful first step is to present your baby with a spoon pre-loaded with something that he is accustomed to eating. If he seems reluctant to take the spoon in his hand, try, with his permission, touching it gently to his lips, then withdrawing it a little and watching for his response. Modeling the behavior for him by putting the spoon in your own mouth may also be beneficial. If there is concern about gagging or the possibility of choking, or if the reason for the change is that he has begun showing aversive behavior toward the spoon, then firm food strips, food popsicles, frozen straws, and/or a silicone feeder, used under the guidance of a feeding therapist, may be a better option. The aim is to show him that that he can feed himself, interfering as little as possible and allowing him to make his own discoveries. This will provide him with a springboard to begin developing a strong self-feeding skill base.

> We discovered ABLW when our son was almost a year old and really struggling to make the transition to solids. We felt a bit helpless and unsure of the best path forward, but this approach, and our therapist's support, truly helped us turn things around. It gave Levi ownership over the process.
>
> Alyssa and Ben, parents of Levi,
> who didn't take well to spoon feeding

Slow progress

It's very likely that your baby won't eat very much—or even anything at all—for the first few weeks of ABLW. Some babies take longer than others to develop the necessary skills, so patience is crucial. Others simply show no interest in food, even though they could pick it up if they wanted to. This can be because of previous negative experiences of eating, perhaps caused by physical discomfort (reflux, for example), unpleasant tastes or overfeeding, or they may simply not be developmentally ready to begin. It's important to be flexible rather than feeling you have to follow a rigid plan. For example, some babies are more accepting, at first, of drinking liquids from an open cup than of beginning with food strips or mashes. Pressuring a baby who is not ready to eat almost invariably has a negative effect and results in his eating even less—or possibly refusing to engage with food altogether. The key is to be responsive and not rush him if he is not ready to take this step.

Your baby will be more willing to explore and taste foods if he's alert and calm than if he's sleepy or hungry. If he shows clear signs of being upset the minute you put him in his high chair, check that you haven't overlooked some of the basics.

- Is he uncomfortable? Can you add some padding to the chair? Does he need his diaper changed?

- Is he tired and in need of a nap?

- Does he feel worried or insecure? It may be worth sitting him on your lap for a few sessions, to help him feel safe in this new experience. You could also try tucking something soft around him, to help him balance and so that he doesn't feel lost.

- Does he need a milk feed? When first starting solid foods, it's a good idea to make sure he *doesn't* have an empty belly when he comes to the table because he hasn't yet learned that solid food can solve his hunger—and, of course, he doesn't yet have the skills to eat it, either.

If your baby is reluctant to try new foods, he may benefit from pairing a familiar food with one that is unfamiliar, for example, dipping a carrot strip (known) into some hummus (new). You could also experiment with presenting a food he likes in a different way, such as offering him a piece of banana on a fork instead of mashed on a spoon. This will help him learn that it's worth tasting what appears to be a new food because it might turn out to be good.

Above all, avoid tricking your baby. He should always feel that he can trust you, and you risk jeopardizing that trust if you mislead him into eating or drinking something he doesn't want. For example, giving him a favorite smoothie laced with something he dislikes is more likely to lead to his refusing the smoothie than deciding he likes the disliked food after all. A similar ploy, recommended by some health professionals, is to hide a bitter vegetable, such as spinach, in a sweet food such as a brownie. Even if it "works," all it's done is teach the baby to eat brownies, not given him a liking for spinach. Sensitive babies can be like food detectives and easily spot when a familiar food has been altered in taste. It's not worth the risk of your baby rejecting a liked food just to see if you can fool him into eating something he would otherwise refuse. It's much better to be honest and, by continuing to offer liked, unliked, and new foods, allow him to expand his repertoire in his own time.

Transitioning to independent and safe self-feeding is a marathon, not a sprint. Sometimes all that's needed is to wait a few more weeks, keeping an eye out for readiness cues, like your baby taking more of his toys to his mouth, or reaching toward what you are eating, to help you determine when to have another go. If you are patient, and respond to his feeding behavior, he will get to where he needs to be.

> ABLW was a miracle for us. At first we were hugely skeptical but it worked wonders, and Sam is now an incredible eater. We are so thankful that we found this approach and persevered, through our initial hesitancy, to follow through with it.
>
> Ben and Maureen, parents of Sam, born at 26 weeks' gestation

THEODORA'S STORY

Jill's account

THEODORA'S HISTORY

Theodora is her parents' second daughter. Her older sister, while she had no significant medical history, was reported to be a picky eater. Theodora was found to have a shortened muscle in one side of her neck (torticollis) and struggled with feeding from birth. Her mom experienced high blood pressure after their discharge from the hospital, needed to be readmitted the day they arrived home, and was put on medication. While she initially attempted a combination of breast- and bottle feeding, dealing with the stress of her high blood pressure put an end to the breastfeeding.

When Theodora was 2 months old, her mom mentioned to the pediatrician that she was choking during bottle feeding. She was referred for a fiberoptic endoscopic evaluation of swallowing (FEES), the results of which indicated that she was aspirating liquid into her lungs with "every sip" and was even sometimes doing so silently—that is, milk was entering her airway and she was showing no response. The decision was made to thicken her feeds to a honey-type consistency (IDDSI level 3) and the speech pathologist at the hospital recommended adding a half-oatmeal, half-rice-cereal mixture to her bottles of formula. After the introduction of this cereal combination, Theodora broke out in eczema all over her body and started having gas pains and "blow-out" diapers. The rice cereal was deemed to be the cause, so she continued with just oatmeal added to her bottles.

Theodora's digestive symptoms and eczema persisted and, when she was 11 weeks old, her medical team experimented with four different infant formulas in an effort to relieve them.

Unfortunately, Theodora had difficulty tolerating any of them. She was subsequently diagnosed with a milk protein allergy and switched to a hydrolysate formula. She was also prescribed two medications to treat reflux. A second FEES when she was 5 months old showed little improvement, and she continued to require feeds of a honey-type consistency.

THEODORA'S FEEDING THERAPY INTERVENTION AND PROGRESS

I evaluated Theodora for the first time when she was 4 months old, as part of a developmental team that included a developmental therapist, physical therapist, and dietitian. By now she was finishing her thickened bottles in about 5 minutes but was very gassy and uncomfortable. She would produce big burps and, reportedly, foul-smelling gas. During the evaluation, she was extremely fussy and uncomfortable, to the point where her parents would frequently have to hold and console her and we were unable to handle her. Having seen how distressed Theodora was, the dietitian and I agreed that the oatmeal that was being used to thicken her formula feeds should immediately be switched to a hypoallergenic thickener.

We began active feeding therapy when Theodora was 5 months old. Our initial sessions were in person, but, after three months, they became virtual. By the time therapy started, the combination of the new thickener and the reflux medications was working, and Theodora was clearly feeling much better. Her gross motor skills had begun to show improvement and bottle feedings were more pleasant for both her and her parents. Immediately after our first therapy session, she had her second FEES, which showed that she was continuing to aspirate liquids thinner than a nectar consistency (IDDSI level 2), so she would need to remain on thickened fluids. At around this time there were signs that, as a result of the restricted head movements caused by the torticollis, she might be developing a flattened area on her skull, so she started wearing a helmet to help correct this and maintain the shape of her head. She continued to wear the helmet until 7 months.

We started with adapted BLW as soon as Theodora turned 6 months. At that point she was still receiving physical therapy aimed at working on body symmetry and transitional movements, but she was able to sit with support in a high chair. We tried applesauce on a pre-loaded spoon as her first food: After an initial gag response she brought the spoon to her mouth twice more and even gnawed on it. From there we worked mainly on hand-to-mouth skills, using slightly thickened commercial Stage 2 purees presented on a pre-loaded spoon or in a silicone feeder. We also tried a frozen banana in the feeder, which Theodora really liked. We had to be cautious, as if she bit down firmly, too much food would come out at once, causing her to gag. We avoided popsicles, since they would have melted into a thin liquid, possibly leading to aspiration.

We quickly moved to putting soft solids, like butternut squash and banana, in the feeder, which Theodora had enough jaw strength to extract. We also began some open-cup drinking of purees thickened to a honey-type consistency. She swiftly graduated to eating small soft solid pieces, such as banana, off a fork, and could manage foods like strawberries, which are harder to break down, in the feeder. By 8 months she could use a raking gesture to pick up small pieces of, for example, avocado and a meltable snack food, and she could gnaw on a strip of meat such as pork roast. She had also learned to drink slightly thinned almond milk yogurt from a therapeutic straw cup without help.

By 9 months, Theodora had developed a pincer grasp for

picking up small pieces and was using her tongue to move food effectively to her lateral gum surfaces for chewing. She quickly progressed to table foods such as meatballs, muffins, waffles, chicken thighs, potato, broccoli, and cod. She would sometimes overstuff her mouth if she had too much food in front of her at once, but she generally managed very well. At around this time she had her first experience of cow's milk yogurt and promptly vomited. Shortly afterward she was found to be intolerant to cow dairy and allergic to peanut and egg, which limited what we could offer her, so we had to work closely with the dietitian. Luckily, we later found out that she could digest egg and dairy without a reaction when they were baked into composite foods.

Between 9 and 12 months, Theodora's parents and I worked with Theodora on jaw grading and biting strength, as well as chewing. We used large foods, like a partially peeled apple, for gnawing, and meltable solids for biting practice. Theodora imitated "bite and pull" with resistive toast strips after her mom modeled the action, although she pushed out the bitten-off pieces with her tongue. From the age of 1 year, a big part of her therapy focused on thinning the consistency of her drinks so that eventually she would be able to manage both milk and water without any thickening. Her mom did this very gradually, to ensure safety, while at the same time weaning her from the bottle to the open cup and straw cup.

At 12 months, Theodora was walking independently. She no longer needed physical therapy or her reflux medications and was sharing all her family's foods, in strips and pieces, as well as gnawing on large foods. Her skills with solid foods were excellent, so we focused on utensil use and open-cup drinking and on helping her to pace herself with straw drinking. She transitioned from formula to a milk made from pea protein, which her mom experimented with to create a nectar consistency (IDDSI level 2), so that Theodora could drink it safely. She eventually graduated to thin liquids and outgrew her allergies by her second birthday. Her parents continue to collaborate with Theodora's pediatrician as to when and if she will undergo a repeat FEES now that she is drinking thin liquids.

DISCUSSION

Theodora's progress has been particularly heartening. Her family was really struggling at the onset of therapy and Theodora was very fussy and uncomfortable as a young baby. As we worked on responsive bottle feeding, made dietary changes in conjunction with the dietitian, and helped Theodora find a team that could manage her medical issues, she became a different baby. Swapping the oatmeal for the hypoallergenic thickener was a particular breakthrough, allowing her to become a happy, social, and engaging little girl, simply because she was no longer in pain.

I think Theodora's parents were initially skeptical about ABLW, but we introduced solid foods very gradually to ensure that she developed good chewing skills. We were all delighted when, at one year, she could bite off pieces from a whole peeled apple, chew them thoroughly, and swallow them safely. Her mom also felt that Theodora's enthusiastic eating was influencing her older, picky-eating sister to be more adventurous.

It seemed to me that the stress experienced by the family over Theodora's difficulty with managing thin liquids was overwhelming. Her mom followed the IDDSI guidelines scrupulously, to make sure that Theodora's liquids were the correct consistency to allow her to stay safe. The fact that she was such a great eater of solid foods likely helped strengthen her swallow and enabled her to become confident with both eating and drinking. I also believe that using ABLW helped to reduce the pressure over thin liquids and allow Theodora the space to develop her other eating skills.

Theodora's mom's perspective

I was terrified at the prospect of Theodora starting solid foods. Our baby couldn't drink clear water without choking, so how on earth was she going to handle a piece of toast?! It really frightened me at first and I'm so grateful we were able to take things slowly—first with pre-loaded spoons, and then longer strips of food Theodora could gnaw at—because it helped me get comfortable. I also found it really helpful to learn about a baby's gag reflex being closer to the front of her tongue than an adult's, and to have someone knowledgeable coach me through the gagging and explain which gags had more to do with Theodora exploring a new food texture, rather than her actually struggling with the food. I remember being very stressed and sad when she tried green beans for the first time and gagged so hard she threw up a little. But I also remember how proud I was when she took a whole apple or whole pear from me for the first time and was able to hold, bite, manipulate, and chew it. It was astonishing to see my little baby actually able to feed herself without choking. It was so empowering and satisfying to see her confidently eating, after watching her suffer, and looking helplessly into her watery eyes when she would choke on her water.

I've been shocked by Theodora's confidence and skill in manipulating food. She has much better coordination than I would have imagined. I think she is more skilled in knowing how to manipulate food than my four-year-old. I would have panicked if my older daughter ate grapes or raisins at two years, but Theodora eats these foods all the time and handles them like a pro. There are now very few fruits that I need to cut for her, as she has learned how to bite and chew—and how to spit out when she takes in more food than she can handle (as she sometimes does with cheese). I'm also constantly surprised by her confidence. She often pushes me away and insists on doing things on her own—especially eating food. She doesn't hesitate: She'll grab a slice of pizza or a chicken leg, or an entire palmful of pasta, and she very successfully eats her meals. She never asks for any help, only for more food. She's also now an expert with her fork and spoon. In fact, I was chuckling the other day because she insisted on eating her meat with a spoon but her rice with a fork. Hey—it's not what I would have done, but she ate her whole meal with no trouble! And the mess is slowly getting less, as well. She's drinking well, too. This past Thanksgiving we were all grateful that she can now drink water.

Our baby's feeding issues had a huge impact on the way we approach food in our home. I used a traditional approach in feeding our elder daughter. I made her homemade organic baby fruit purees and now, as we approach her fifth birthday, she is a painfully picky eater. It impacts our family's choices on where we can order out from. She only really eats bread, cheese, fruit, and pasta. Meanwhile, the baby-led weaning approach we used with our youngest has her eating just about anything we present. She'll consistently eat whatever main meal is on the table, and she even eats foods that I don't, like salmon. Until we met Jill we'd always resort to separate meals for our elder daughter and for ourselves, but once we began doing ABLW, we started to approach meals more as a full family experience. We would put the food on platters and bowls on the table and allow both girls to choose from everything we were having. This positively impacted our picky daughter in a lot of ways because, with a low-pressure exposure to the foods, she would sometimes choose to try new things. Also, I am very lucky that I have been able to work from home and can eat lunch together with my girls most days. Modeling what I'm eating has really impacted the foods Theodora is open to eating. If it's not on her plate but it is on mine, she's probably going to try it! She hates being left out and always wants what others around her have.

It's very apparent that eating is a much different experience for both our daughters. My oldest sees it as a chore, and it's always a struggle to get her to eat that one more bite. Our youngest, however, eats with joy, pleasure, and gusto! I remember when Theodora was about 22 months we made a big salad and left it on the table. Theodora reached in and was eating tomatoes out of the bowl. I couldn't believe it: Her sister would never have done that and she was four years old! Now that she can speak, Theodora will say that things are yummy and ask for more, and she really enjoys her meals. It brings me huge joy—that this child who struggled so much can not only eat but that she enjoys eating so much. It makes me so excited to make new foods for her to try.

CONCLUSION

That's it—you've reached the end of this book! We hope you've enjoyed it, but above all we hope we've succeeded in giving you the information you need to support a baby who faces feeding and eating challenges to become a safe and competent self-feeder and to enjoy discovering and eating solid foods.

The philosophy that underpins ABLW encompasses not just nutritional issues and physical development, but wider issues of autonomy and self-determination. It's about respect for all babies, and the children and adults they will grow into. We consider the experience of eating to be at least as important for a child's relationship with food as the food itself, and that this matters from the very beginning. For too long, discussions of infant feeding have focused on the "what" and "when" of solid foods, with very little attention being paid to the "how"—especially for babies facing feeding challenges. We are confident that, through their ABLW journey, the babies you may care for will be primed for a lifelong love of food.

As you'll have grasped if you've read this far, we aren't against the use of spoons and purees; we just don't go along with the idea that babies—whether typically developing or facing feeding challenges—need to have all their food pureed or be fed by someone else. We think they deserve to be recognized for what they *can* do, not held back because of what they can't yet manage. It's our belief that with the right support, every baby has the potential to become a confident and intuitive eater—and that their parents and caregivers can be empowered and enabled to provide that support.

When BLW first came on the scene, it was regarded by many as a feeding fad that they imagined would quickly disappear. But they reckoned without the thousands of parents who understood it as something fundamentally right, and who quickly discovered the benefits it offered to them and their families. The BLW approach has achieved the level of popularity it has today because of the enthusiasm of parents and the advocacy of the few health professionals who were prepared to think outside the box.

ABLW is in a similar position now to where BLW was fifteen years ago. Having initially been greeted with dismay and skepticism, it is rapidly gaining ground as an accepted and therapeutic approach to transitioning to solid foods for babies with a vast range of health and developmental challenges. We see this book as a way to sustain and accelerate this revolution, among both parents and those who advise them. If you're already on board, be sure to spread the word and share your enthusiasm with others. And if you're intrigued but hesitating—come on in! It's time to involve all babies in decisions about their feeding journey.

APPENDIX

Therapists who may be involved in an individual baby's care

There are a number of therapists whose individual expertise extends beyond the realm of the transition to solid foods but overlaps in this critical area.

Lactation Consultant

An International Board-Certified Lactation Consultant (IBCLC)'s area of expertise is in education and clinical management related to breastfeeding. They are able to provide information and support around establishing a milk supply, positioning and latching a baby on to the breast, use of pumps to express milk, management of breastfeeding issues (such as pain and discomfort), use of special breastfeeding devices (such as a supplemental nursing system), and assessing milk transfer.

Not all practitioners who use the title lactation consultant are IBCLC-qualified, which means their practice is not regulated by the International Board of Lactation Consultant Examiners (IBCLE). On the other hand, there are IBCLCs whose work extends more widely, meaning that they identify themselves by another title—midwife, for example. It's worth seeking out someone who has the international qualification if you want to be sure they have a high level of education and experience.

Dietitian

A registered pediatric dietitian's area of expertise is in supporting parents and professional colleagues to manage the nutritional needs, weight, and growth of babies and children. They may recommend what the components of the child's diet should be and suggest ideas for specific foods and/or supplements that will enhance macro- and micronutrient intake. They will also be able to make dietary recommendations for issues such as reflux and constipation. They may have additional expertise in weaning babies from reliance on tube feeding, helping to ensure continued and appropriate nourishment while the baby is transitioning to oral feedings.

A dietitian is not the same as a nutritionist. While the work of both revolves around food, most nutritionists are not trained to offer support in situations where the ability to eat or digest food is compromised or when the individual has complex medical needs. A registered dietitian is qualified to provide medical nutrition therapy (MNT) in situations where a patient has a specific diagnosis, such as weight-faltering, where dietary modifications (for example, a high-calorie, high-protein diet) are needed. Registered dietitians have to meet specific educational and clinical guidelines and pass a board exam in order to use that title. In the US, they are credentialed by the Commission on Dietetic Registration (CDR) and are members of the Academy of Nutrition and Dietetics (AND).

Physical therapist (PT)

The pediatric physical therapist's expertise is in the area of balance, posture, and gross (large) motor skills, such as rolling, sitting, crawling, and walking. They will be able to evaluate and treat babies who may have bony, muscular, or neurological issues or impaired or delayed development. They will work and advise on ways to improve core strength, trunk control, range of motion, and movement patterns to help babies reach their gross motor milestones and achieve their full potential. They may work on those skills using positioning, exercises, a therapy ball and/or bench sitting, as well as recreational activities like swimming. Physical therapists have many years of training, with some being doctors of physical therapy. In the US, physical therapists need to be licensed and are governed by the American Physical Therapy Association (APTA).

Developmental therapist (DT)

A developmental therapist (sometimes called a developmental specialist or early childhood special educator [ECSE]) has training in typical and atypical development and can evaluate and provide intervention techniques to families in the areas of cognition, play, speech and language, adaptive skills, social-emotional development, and gross motor and fine motor skills. They work mainly through play and caregiver coaching to encourage skill development. DTs may also be able to assist families in managing issues like behavior and difficulty sleeping. Some specialize in working with children with vision loss or deafness. The educational requirements for DTs vary by individual state, but they minimally hold a bachelor's degree in early childhood education or a related field. Certification and licensure requirements for DTs also vary from state to state; most require additional infant/toddler coursework to become credentialed as an early intervention developmental therapist.

Speech-language pathologist (SLP)

The pediatric speech-language pathologist's area of expertise is more wide-ranging than the title suggests. It covers verbal and nonverbal communication, feeding and swallowing, and voice. When therapy is needed from birth, speech pathologists work on feeding skills first, gradually transitioning to a focus on communication skills as the baby develops. They spend time in neonatal intensive care units, assisting with the feeding of pre-term babies by breast and bottle, and with the transition from tube to oral feedings.

SLPs work intensively with babies who have diagnoses that affect how they eat, using a range of therapeutic techniques to stimulate the use and development of muscles related to breathing, feeding, and speech, usually as lead feeding therapist. They may also be part of a team with radiologists, carrying out detailed assessments of swallowing and recommending the safest food and liquid consistencies for babies whose swallowing ability is compromised. In cases where complementary feeding brings challenges, the SLP will demonstrate and advise on the sizes, shapes, and textures of food that will enhance chewing and swallowing.

Speech-language pathologists also evaluate and treat babies with communication difficulties, showing parents ways to facilitate understanding of language, and develop expressive communication skills through play, storytelling, and songs, as well as sign language and specialist communicative devices. They are required to complete a master's degree, and many are now achieving clinical doctorates in speech-language pathology. In the US, SLPs require licensure; their regulatory organization is the American Speech-Language-Hearing Association (ASHA).

Occupational therapist (OT)

The pediatric occupational therapist's expertise is in general development, with a focus on self-care, fine motor skills, and sensory integration. The OT will help babies with everyday activities, such as grasping toys, working on fine and visual motor skills—for example, visual tracking and eye-hand coordination—through play and fun activities. An OT can collaborate with a caregiver on strategies to make daily routines easier, including bathing, dressing, diapering, and play. They may also recommend ways for parents and caregivers to calm an anxious or disorganized baby around mealtime, through techniques such as soothing massage or gentle swinging.

Because eating is a major occupation, many OTs specialize in feeding issues, assisting with positioning for feeding and adaptive seating systems. OTs are equipped to take on the role of lead feeding therapist; where that role is assumed by the speech-language pathologist, the OT can nevertheless be instrumental in teaching techniques that other therapists—and the baby's caregivers—can use to help him learn more refined movements for feeding. They can work on utensil use and share strategies and techniques for working with babies who are unusually sensitive to textures, odors or sounds. They may help to desensitize a child who does not cope well with variations in texture (generally and with food) through gentle, controlled exposure.

Occupational therapists must have a master's degree and some go on to obtain an occupational therapy doctorate. They are required to be licensed, and they are regulated by the American Occupational Therapy Association (AOTA).

NOTES

Preface

1. Solid Starts' #FingerFoodFirst campaign (launching January 2023) aims to educate professionals working in pediatrics on the benefits of the early introduction of finger foods, solidstarts.com; Instagram: @solidstarts.

Chapter 1

1. R. S. Corruccini, *How Anthropology Informs the Orthodontic Diagnosis of Malocclusions' Causes* (Lewiston, NY: Edwin Mellen Press, 1999).

2. D. W. Sellen, "Evolution of Infant and Young Child Feeding: Implications for Contemporary Public Health," *Annual Review of Nutrition* 27 (2007): 123–48.

3. G. H. Pelto et al., "Premastication: The Second Arm of Infant and Young Child Feeding for Health and Survival?," *Maternal & Child Nutrition* 6, no. 1 (2010): 4–18.

4. E. E. Stevens et al., "A History of Infant Feeding," *Journal of Perinatal Education* 18, no. 2 (2009): 32–39.

5. A. Bentley, *Inventing Baby Food: Taste, Health, and the Industrialization of the American Diet* (Oakland: University of California Press, 2014).

6. "Baby Food Market—Global Industry Analysis," Zion Market Research, zionmarketresearch.com. Accessed April 29, 2022.

7. R. D. Stevenson and J. H. Allaire, "The Development of Normal Feeding and Swallowing," *Pediatric Clinics of North America* 38, no. 6 (1991): 1439–53.

8. I. Zen et al., "Maxillary Arch Dimensions in the First 6 Months of Life and Their Relationship with Pacifier Use," *European Archives of Paediatric Dentistry* 21, no. 3 (2020): 313–19.

9. M. Potock and M. H. Katz, *Responsive Feeding: The Baby-First Guide to Stress-Free Weaning, Healthy Eating, and Mealtime Bonding* (New York: The Experiment, 2022).

10. "Oversight Subcommittee Staff Report Reveals Top Baby Foods Contain Dangerous Levels of Toxic Heavy Metals," House Committee on Oversight and Reform, February 4, 2021, oversight.house.gov.

11. A. Greene, "2011 White Paper: Why White Rice Cereal for Babies Must Go," drgreene.com. Accessed April 29, 2022.

12. N. F. Krebs, "Dietary Zinc and Iron Sources, Physical Growth and Cognitive Development of Breastfed Infants," Supplement, *Journal of Nutrition* 130, no. 2 (2000): 358S–60S.

13. A. I. Eidelman et al., "Breastfeeding and the Use of Human Milk," *Pediatrics* 129, no. 3 (2012): e827–41.

Chapter 2

1. A. I. Eidelman et al., op. cit.

2. "World Health Organization/UNICEF," *Global Strategy for Infant and Young Child Feeding* (Geneva, Switzerland: WHO, 2003).

3. "The Satter division of responsibility in feeding," Ellyn Satter Institute, ellynsatterinstitute.org. Accessed April 29, 2022.

4. "A History of the 100 First Foods Approach to Baby-Led Weaning," *Baby-Led Weaning Made Easy* episode 63, blwpodcast.com.

5. H. Coulthard and A.-M. Sealy, "Play with Your Food! Sensory Play Is Associated with Tasting of Fruits and Vegetables in Preschool Children," *Appetite* 113 (2017): 84–90.

6. F. C. Powell et al., "Food Avoidance in Children. The Influence of Maternal Feeding Practices and Behaviours," *Appetite* 57, no. 3 (2011): 683–92.

7. K. C. Borowitz and S. M. Borowitz, "Feeding Problems in Infants and Children: Assessment and Etiology," *Pediatric Clinics of North America* 65, no. 1 (2018): 59–72.

8. G. Harris and S. Mason, "Are There Sensitive Periods for Food Acceptance in Infancy?," *Current Nutrition Reports* 6, no. 2 (2017): 190–6.

9. A. Brown and M. Lee, "A Descriptive Study Investigating the Use and Nature of Baby-Led Weaning in a UK Sample of Mothers," *Maternal & Child Nutrition* 7, no. 1 (2011): 34–47.

10. A. P. Moore et al., "An Online Survey of Knowledge of the Weaning Guidelines, Advice from Health Visitors and Other Factors That Influence Weaning Timing in UK Mothers," *Maternal & Child Nutrition* 10, no. 3 (2014): 410–21.

11. M. Campeau et al., "The Baby-Led Weaning Method: A Focus on Mealtime Behaviours, Food Acceptance and Fine Motor Skills," *Nutrition Bulletin* 46, no. 4 (2021): 476–85; B. J. Morison et al., "Impact of a Modified Version of Baby-Led Weaning on Dietary Variety and Food Preferences in infants," *Nutrients* 10, no. 8 (2018): 1092.

12. E. Townsend and N. J. Pitchford, "Baby Knows Best? The Impact of Weaning Style on Food Preferences and Body Mass Index in Early Childhood in a Case-Controlled Sample," *BMJ Open* 2, no. 1 (2012): e000298.

13. A. Brown and M. Lee, "Early Influences on Child Satiety Responsiveness: The Role of Weaning Style," *Pediatric Obesity* 10, no. 1 (2015): 57–66.

14. X. Fu, C. A. Conlon et al., "Food Fussiness and Early Feeding Characteristics of Infants Following Baby-Led Weaning and Traditional Spoon feeding in New Zealand: An Internet Survey," *Appetite* 130 (2018): 110–16; R. W. Taylor et al., "Effect of a Baby-Led Approach to Complementary Feeding on Infant Growth and Overweight: A Randomised Clinical Trial," *JAMA Pediatrics* 171, no. 9 (2017): 838–46.

15. A. Brown, "No Difference in Self-Reported Frequency of Choking Between Infants Introduced to Solid Foods Using a Baby-Led Weaning or Traditional Spoon Feeding Approach," *Journal of Human Nutrition and Dietetics* 31, no. 4 (2018); E. Dogan et al., "Baby-Led Complementary Feeding: Randomized Controlled Study," *Pediatrics International* 60, no. 12 (2018): 1073–80; Taylor et al., op. cit.

16. Townsend and Pitchford, op. cit.; Brown and Lee, op. cit.; Taylor et al., op. cit.

17. E. Addessi et al., "Baby-Led Weaning in Italy and Potential Implications for Infant Development," *Appetite*, 164 (2021): 105286; Campeau et al., op. cit.; C. Webber et al., "An Infant-Led Approach to Complementary Feeding Is Positively Associated with Language Development," *Maternal & Child Nutrition* 17, no. 4 (2021): e13206.

18. K. Boyd et al., "Culture, Industrialisation and the Shrinking Human Face: Why Is It Important?," *European Journal of Paediatric Dentistry* 22, no. 1 (2021): 80–82.

19. M. M. Black and F. E. Aboud, "Responsive Feeding Is Embedded in a Theoretical Framework of Responsive Parenting," *Journal of Nutrition* 141, no. 3 (2011): 490–94.

20. "Infant and young child feeding," World Health Organization, June 9, 2021, who.int.

21. "The Satter division of responsibility in feeding," op. cit.

22. The Get Permission Institute, getpermissioninstitute.com. Accessed April 29, 2022.

23. We prefer the term eye-hand to hand-eye because babies' vision comes before movement and drives it. For example, a baby will look at what he wants to pick up before moving his hand toward it.

Chapter 3

1. S. D. Colson et al., "Optimal Positions Triggering Primitive Neonatal Reflexes Stimulating Breastfeeding," *Early Human Development* 84, no.7 (2008): 441–49.

2. R. Alexander et al., *Normal Development of Functional Motor Skills: The First Year of Life* (Tucson, AZ: Therapy Skill Builders, 1993).

3. C. W. Genna et al., "Quantitative Imaging of Tongue Kinematics During Infant Feeding and Adult Swallowing Reveals Highly Conserved Patterns," *Physiological Reports* 9, no. 3 (2021): e14685.

4. S. E. Morris and M. D. Klein, *Pre-Feeding Skills: A Comprehensive Resource for Mealtime Development* (Tucson, AZ: Therapy Skill Builders, 2000).

5. J. L. Miller et al., "Emergence of Oropharyngeal, Laryngeal, and Swallowing Activity in the Developing Fetal Upper Aerodigestive Tract: An Ultrasound Evaluation," *Early Human Development* 71, no. 1 (2003): 61–87.

6. E. M. Wilson and J. R. Green, "The Development of Jaw Motion for Mastication," *Early Human Development* 85, no. 5 (2009): 303–11.

7. E. J. Gibson and A. S. Walker, "Development of Knowledge of Visual-Tactual Affordances of Substance," *Child Development* 55 (1984): 453–60.

8. S. E. Shune and J. B. Moon, "Effects of Age and Non-Oropharyngeal Proprioceptive and Exteroceptive Sensation on the Magnitude of Anticipatory Mouth Opening During Eating," *Journal of Oral Rehabilitation* 43, No. 9 (2016): 662–69.

9. P. G. Meyer, "Tongue lip and jaw differentiation and its relationship to orofacial myofunctional treatment," *International Journal of Orofacial Myology* 26, no. 1 (2008): 38–46.

10. J. A. Mennella et al., "Prenatal and Postnatal Flavor Learning by Human Infants," *Pediatrics* 107, no. 6 (2001): e88.

11. J. Werthmann et al., "Bits and Pieces: Food Texture Influences Food Acceptance in Young Children," *Appetite* 84 (2015): 181–87.

12. M. Gelb and H. Hindin, *Gasp: Airway Health—The Hidden Path to Wellness* (New York: CreateSpace Independent Publishing Platform, 2016).

13. P. Haggard and L. de Boer, "Oral Somatosensory Awareness," *Neuroscience & Biobehavioral Reviews* 47 (2014): 469–84.

14. L. Avivi-Arber et al., "Face Sensorimotor Cortex and its Neuroplasticity Related to Orofacial Sensorimotor Functions," *Archives of Oral Biology*, 56, no. 12 (2011): 1440–65.

15. S. E. Morris and M. D. Klein, op. cit.

16. S. E. Shune et al., "The Effects of Age and Preoral Sensorimotor Cues on Anticipatory Mouth Movement During Swallowing," *Journal of Speech, Language, and Hearing Research* 59, no. 2 (2016): 195–205.

17. A. H. Zachry et al., "Infant Positioning, Baby Gear Use, and Cranial Asymmetry," *Maternal and Child Health Journal* 21, no. 12 (2017): 2229–36.

18. P. Rochat, "Mouthing and Grasping in Neonates: Evidence for the Early Detection of What Hard or Soft Substances Afford for Action," *Infant Behavior & Development* 10, no. 4 (1987): 435–49.

19. A. J. Miller, "Oral and Pharyngeal Reflexes in the Mammalian Nervous System: Their Diverse Range in Complexity and the Pivotal Role of the Tongue," *Critical Reviews in Oral Biology & Medicine* 13, no. 5 (2002): 409–25.

20. A. Brown, "No Difference in Self-Reported Frequency of Choking between Infants Introduced to Solid Foods Using a Baby-Led Weaning or Traditional Spoon Feeding Approach," *Journal of Human Nutrition and Dietetics* 31, no. 4: 496–504 (2018); E. Dogan et al., "Baby-Led Complementary Feeding: Randomized Controlled Study," *Pediatrics International* 60, no. 12 (2018): 1073–80.

Chapter 4

1.   B. R. Carruth et al., "Prevalence of Picky Eaters among Infants and Toddlers and Their Caregivers' Decisions about Offering a New Food," *Journal of the American Dietetic Association* 104, no. 1 (2004): 57–64.

2.   M. A. Podporina et al., "Eating behavior and skills of babies born prematurely at different age periods," *Voprosy Pitaniia* 91, no.1 (2022): 19–26.

3.   M.-C. Chang et al., "Study of Orofacial Function in Preschool Children Born Prematurely," *Children* 9, no. 3 (2022): 360.

4.   C. F. Ross et al., "Parent-Reported Ease of Eating Foods of Different Textures in Young Children with Down Syndrome," *Journal of Texture Studies* 50, no. 5 (2019): 426–33.

5.   K. C. Borowitz and S. M. Borowitz, op. cit.

6.   A. H. Ans et al., "Neurohormonal Regulation of Appetite and Its Relationship with Stress: A Mini Literature Review," *Cureus* 10, no. 7 (2018): e3032.

7.   W. J. Di Scipio et al., "Traumatically Acquired Conditioned Dysphagia in Children," *Annals of Otology, Rhinology and Laryngology* 87, no. 4 (1978): 509–14.

8.   "The IDDSI Framework," International Dysphagia Diet Standardisation Initiative, iddsi.org. Accessed April 29, 2022.

9.   K. Northstone et al., "The Effect of Age of Introduction to Lumpy Solids on Foods Eaten and Reported Feeding Difficulties at 6 and 15 Months," *Journal of Human Nutrition and Dietetics* 14, no. 1 (2001): 43–54.

10. K. Boyd et al., op. cit.

11. C. G. Victora et al., "Breastfeeding in the 21st Century: Epidemiology, Mechanisms, and Lifelong Effect," *The Lancet* 387, no. 10017 (2016): 475–90.

12. "WHO/UNICEF: World Health Organization/UNICEF," *Global Strategy for Infant and Young Child Feeding* (Geneva, Switzerland: WHO, 2003).

13. S. L. Rogers et al., "Relationships between Feeding Problems, Eating Behaviours and Parental Feeding Practices in Children with Down Syndrome: A Cross-Sectional Study," *Journal of Applied Research in Intellectual Disabilities* 35, no. 2 (2022): 596–606.

14. P. Fieldhouse, *Food and Nutrition: Customs and Culture* (London: Chapman & Hall Ltd., 1995).

15. C. E. Snow and D. E. Beals, "Mealtime Talk that Supports Literacy Development," *New Directions for Child and Adolescent Development* 111, no. 51 (2006): 51–66.

16. G. Rapley, "Are Puréed Foods Justified for Infants of 6 Months? What Does the Evidence Tell Us?," *Journal of Health Visiting* 4, no. 6 (2016): 289–95.

17. H. Coulthard et al., "Delayed Introduction of Lumpy Foods to Children During the Complementary Feeding Period Affects Child's Food Acceptance and Feeding at 7 Years of Age," *Maternal and Child Nutrition* 5, no. 1 (2009): 75–85.

18. K. Boyd et al., op. cit.

19. B. J. Morison et al., op. cit.; R. W. Taylor et al., op. cit.

20. X. Fu et al., "Food Fussiness and Early Feeding Characteristics of Infants Following Baby-Led Weaning and Traditional Spoon Feeding in New Zealand: An Internet Survey," *Appetite* 130 (2018): 110–16.

21. G. Rapley, "Is Spoon Feeding Justified for Infants of 6 Months? What Does the Evidence Tell Us?," *Journal of Health Visiting* 4, no. 8 (2016): 414–19.

Chapter 5

1.   Early Intervention is the name of a publicly funded program that provides therapeutic services for 0–3-year-olds who have developmental delays and disabilities. In most cases, families whose child is eligible can receive this support for free or at reduced cost. The program exists in every state in the USA, although the range of services and the way they are implemented varies from state to state; see "What Is 'Early Intervention'?," Centers for Disease Control and Prevention, cdc.gov.

2.   D. C. Bahr, *Nobody Ever Told Me (or My Mother) That!: Everything from Bottles and Breathing to Healthy Speech Development* (Arlington, TX: Sensory World, 2010).

3.   R. Merkel-Walsh and L. L. Overland, *A Sensory Motor Approach to Feeding* (Charleston, SC: TalkTools, 2013); R. Merkel-Walsh and L. L. Overland, *Functional Assessment and Remediation of TOTs (Tethered Oral Tissues)* (Charleston, SC: TalkTools, 2018).

4.   Some parents and professionals may find an online course such as the Tummy Time! Method useful: tummytimemethod.com.

5.   C. Guilleminault and Y.-S. Huang, "From Oral Facial Dysfunction to Dysmorphism and the Onset of Pediatric OSA," *Sleep Medicine Reviews* 40 (2018): 203–14.

6.   R. Merkel-Walsh and L. L. Overland, op. cit.

7.   Ibid.

8.   Ibid.

Chapter 6

1.   For a discussion of why molded seats are not a good idea; see blog.dinopt.com/bumbo-is-a-no-go.

2.   There are a number of excellent high chairs available at the time of writing. Some examples that work particularly well for the neurodiverse population are the Stokke Tripp Trapp, Nomi, Abiie Beyond, and Oxo Tot Sprout, all of which facilitate good positioning of the trunk and pelvis and come with adjustable footrests.

3.   For example, the High Chair Helper from TalkTools; see talktools.com.

Chapter 7

1. "Foods and Drinks for 6 to 24 Month Olds," Centers for Disease Control and Prevention, cdc.gov. Accessed April 29, 2022.

2. S. D. Brown and G. Harris, "A Theoretical Proposal for a Perceptually Driven, Food-Based Disgust That Can Influence Food Acceptance During Early Childhood," *International Journal of Child Health and Nutrition* 1, no. 1 (2012): 1–10.

3. F. Zampollo et al., "Food Plating Preferences of Children: The Importance of Presentation on Desire for Diversity," *Acta Paediatrica* 101, no. 1 (2012): 61–66.

4. K. Northstone et al., "The Effect of Age of Introduction to Lumpy Solids on Foods Eaten and Reported Feeding Difficulties at 6 and 15 Months," *Journal of Human Nutrition and Dietetics* 14, no. 1 (2001): 43–54.

5. L. Ferrara et al., "Short-Term Effects of Cold Liquids on the Pharyngeal Swallow in Pre-Term Infants with Dysphagia: A Pilot Study," *Dysphagia* 33, no. 5 (2018): 593–601.

6. "The IDDSI Framework," op. cit.

Chapter 8

1. M. D. Klein, *Anxious Eaters, Anxious Mealtimes: Practical and Compassionate Strategies for Mealtime Peace* (Bloomington, IN: Archway Publishing, 2019).

2. The Get Permission Institute, op. cit.

3. "The IDDSI Framework," op. cit.

4. At the time of writing, TalkTools is the best source for therapeutic straws; see talktools.com.

5. K. A. Toomey and E. S. Ross, "SOS Approach to Feeding," *Perspectives on Swallowing and Swallowing Disorders* 20, no. 3 (2011): 82–87; see also sosapproachtofeeding.com.

6. C. Fraker et al., *Food Chaining: The Proven 6-Step Plan to Stop Picky Eating, Solve Feeding Problems, and Expand Your Child's Diet* (Philadelphia: Da Capo Press, 2007).

7. R. Merkel-Walsh and L. L. Overland, op. cit.

Chapter 9

1. M. D. Klein, op. cit.

RESOURCES

WEBSITES AND SOCIAL MEDIA

Baby-led weaning is all over the internet these days. We have listed just a few of the resources that you may find useful but there are many others. Please note that we do not necessarily endorse everything that is suggested by the individuals and organizations listed here but we consider that their approach is generally in line with ours.

General information about BLW

Jill Rabin: jillrabin.com

Gill Rapley: rapleyweaning.com

Gill Rapley and Tracey Murkett: allaboutblw.co.uk

Katie Ferraro: fortifiedfam.com

Solid Starts: solidstarts.com

Untethered Podcast—interview with Jill Rabin: untetheredpodcast
.com/ 2019/12/30/episode-31-jill-rabin-m-s-ccc-slp-l-ibclc

The Sleep Sessions—interview with Gill Rapley: podcasts.apple.com/
us/podcast/meet-the-expert-gill-rapley-author-of-baby-led-
weaning/id1497905903?i=1000473415640

Baby-Led Weaning Made Easy (Katie Ferraro)—several interviews with
Jill Rabin and/or Gill Rapley: blwpodcast.com, plus courses on BLW

Real Food Littles—online course on BLW: realfoodlittles.com

Down Syndrome Resource Foundation: dsrf.org/
programs-&-resources/the-lowdown-podcast/
the-lowdown,-episode-5-4

INFORMATION FOR PARENTS

Feeding and general development

Ages and Stages—Diane Bahr: agesandstages.net

Baby Foode (recipes and food ideas): babyfoode.com

Baby-Led Weaning Made Easy—Katie Ferraro: blwpodcast.com

Cate Fox, dietitian (specialist for Prader-Willi syndrome): catefoxdietitian.com

Chicago Feeding Group: chicagofeedinggroup.org

Extreme Picky Eating—Jenny McGlothlin and Katja Rowell: extremepickyeating.com

Feeding Matters (Pediatric Feeding Disorder): feedingmatters.org

Happy Little Tummies—Amy Manojlovski: happylittletummies.com

Mama and Sweet Pea Nutrition—Meghan McMillin: mamaandsweetpeanutrition.com

New Ways Nutrition—Renae D'Andrea: newwaysnutrition.com

SOS Approach to Feeding—Dr. Kay Toomey and colleagues: sosapproachtofeeding.com

Super Healthy Kids (recipes and food ideas): superhealthykids.com

The Feeding Doctor—Dr. Katja Rowell: thefeedingdoctor.com

Tummy Time! Method—Michelle Emmanuel: tummytimemethod.com

T21 Mom (Focus on challenges such as in Down syndrome): t21mom.com

Instagram: instagram.com

@jillrabinablw
@ableappetites/@ableappetites.esp
@babyledweanteam
@catefoxdietitian
@feedingtinybellies
@healthy.mom.healthy.kids
@msdawnslp
@solidstarts/@solidstartsespanol
@tummytimemethod

Feeding-related equipment

Please note that we are not seeking to promote specific brands, or to advocate all the products in their ranges; this is simply a nonexhaustive list of resources available at the time of writing that may be useful for parents and professionals seeking to implement ABLW.

Tripp Trapp high chair: stokke.com

Nomi high chair: evomove.com

Abiie high chair: abiie.com

Oxo Sprout high chair: oxo.com

Baby Cup (open cup suitable 6-months plus): babycup.co.uk/
physical-stores/categories/united-states

Avanchy (sustainable baby dishware): avanchy.com

EZPZ (cups and utensils suitable 6-months plus): ezpzfun.com

Numnum (Gootensil pre-spoons): numnumbaby.us

Support related to specific conditions

There are many different organizations that offer support and information for the families of babies who have a specific diagnosis. These are just a few of them.

American Cleft Palate-Craniofacial Association: acpa-cpf.org

Cleft Lip and Palate Foundation of Smiles: cleftsmile.org

Down Syndrome Resource Foundation: dsrf.org

Global Down Syndrome Foundation: globaldownsyndrome.org

EA/TEF Child and Family Support Connection (Esophageal Atresia and Tracheoesophageal Fistula): eatef.org

Hand to Hold (NICU babies): handtohold.org

NICU Helping Hands: nicuhelpinghands.org

Noonan Syndrome Foundation: teamnoonan.org

Prader-Willi Syndrome Association: pwsausa.org

Williams Syndrome Association: williams-syndrome.org

Resources for professionals

Ages and Stages—Diane Bahr: agesandstages.net

Alphabet Soup—Lori Overland and colleagues:
alphabetsoupomtherapy.com

Chicago Feeding Group—Stephanie Cohen, Karen Dilfer, and Risa Nasatir: chicagofeedinggroup.org

Extreme Picky Eating—Jenny McGlothlin and Katja Rowell: extremepickyeating.com

First Bite—Michelle Dawson and Erin Forward: firstbite.fireside.fm/

Get Permission Institute—Marsha Dunn Klein and colleagues: getpermissioninstitute.com

International Starting Solids Network—Jessica Coll: networks.jessicacoll.com; healthyinstitute.com

Feeding Matters (Pediatric Feeding Disorder): feedingmatters.org

Professor Amy Brown (research on BLW): professoramybrown.co.uk

Responsive Feeding Pro—Jo Cormack and colleagues: responsivefeedingpro.com

Responsive Feeding Therapy—Jenny McGlothlin, Katja Rowell, and Grace Wong responsivefeedingtherapy.com

SOS Approach to Feeding—Dr. Kay Toomey and colleagues: sosapproachtofeeding.com

TalkTools (courses, conferences, therapy tools): talktools.com

Tummy Time! Method—Michelle Emmanuel: tummytimemethod.com

ARK Therapeutic (therapy tools): arktherapeutic.com

Chewy Tubes (therapy tools): chewytubes.com

FURTHER READING: BOOKS AND PUBLICATIONS

Formula feeding, complementary feeding, and the baby food industry

Bentley, A. *Inventing Baby Food: Taste, Health, and the Industrialization of the American Diet*. Oakland: University of California Press, 2014.

Brown, A. *Why Starting Solids Matters*. London: Pinter & Martin, 2017.

Palmer, G. *Complementary Feeding: Nutrition, Culture and Politics*. London: Pinter & Martin, 2011.

Baby-led weaning and cooking for families

Rapley, Gill. *Baby-Led Weaning: The Essential Guide—How to Introduce Solid Foods and Help Your Baby to Grow Up a Happy and Confident Eater, Completely Updated and Expanded Tenth Anniversary Edition.* New York: The Experiment, 2019.

Rapley, Gill, and Tracey Murkett. *The Baby-Led Weaning Cookbook: Delicious Recipes That Will Help Your Baby Learn to Eat Solid Foods—and That the Whole Family Will Enjoy.* New York: The Experiment, 2011.

Rapley, Gill, and Tracey Murkett. *The Baby-Led Weaning Cookbook, Volume 2: 99 More No-Stress Recipes for the Whole Family.* New York: The Experiment, 2019.

Burton, Dreena. *Plant-Powered Families—Over 100 Kid-Tested, Whole-Foods Vegan Recipes.* Dallas: BenBella Books, 2015.

Greene, Alan R. *Feeding Baby Green: The Earth-Friendly Program for Healthy, Safe Nutrition During Pregnancy, Childhood, and Beyond.* San Francisco: Jossey-Bass, 2009.

Lair, Cynthia. *Feeding the Whole Family: Cooking with Whole Foods: More than 200 Recipes for Babies, Young Children, and Their Parents.* Seattle: Sasquatch Books, 2016.

Schilling, Leslie, and Wendy Jo Peterson. *Born to Eat: Whole, Healthy Foods from Baby's First Bite.* New York: Skyhorse Publishing, 2017.

Sunog, Ron. *Eat The Eight: Preventing Food Allergy with Food and the Imperfect Art of Medicine.* San Francisco: The Nasiona, 2019.

Feeding babies and children with feeding challenges

Bahr, Diane. *Nobody Ever Told Me (or My Mother) That!: Everything from Bottles and Breathing to Healthy Speech Development.* Pensauken, NJ: BookBaby, 2011.

Cullen, E. G., ed. *Breastfeeding & Down Syndrome: A Comprehensive Guide for Mothers and Medical Professionals.* Down Syndrome Pregnancy, 2019.

Fraker, C. et al. *Food Chaining: The Proven 6-Step Plan to Stop Picky Eating, Solve Feeding Problems and Expand Your Child's Diet.* Boston: Da Capo Press, 2007.

Klein, M. D. *Anxious Eaters, Anxious Mealtimes: Practical and Compassionate Strategies for Mealtime Peace.* London: Archway Publishing, 2019.

McGlothlin, J. and K. Rowell. *Helping Your Child With Extremely Picky Eating: A Step-by-Step Guide for Overcoming Selective Eating, Food Aversion, and Feeding Disorders.* Oakland, CA: New Harbinger, 2015.

Morris, S. E. and M. D. Klein. *Pre-Feeding Skills: A Comprehensive Resource for Mealtime Development,* 2nd ed. Austin, TX: Pro-Ed, 2000.

Overland, L. and R. Merkel-Walsh. *A Sensory Motor Approach to Feeding.* Charleston, SC: TalkTools,2013.

Rowell, K. et al. *Responsive Feeding Therapy: Values and Practice.* White Paper available to download at responsivefeedingpro.com/wp-content/uploads/2021/08/WP.RFpro_.v1-1.pdf.

Watson Genna, K. *Supporting Sucking Skills in Breastfeeding Infants,* 3rd ed. Burlington, MA: Jones and Bartlett Learning, 2017.

General interest

Lin, Steven. *The Dental Diet: The Surprising Link between Your Teeth, Real Food, and Life-Changing Natural Health.* San Diego: Hay House, 2019.

Sole-Smith, Virginia. *The Eating Instinct: Food Culture, Body Image, and Guilt in America.* New York: Henry Holt and Company, 2020.

IMAGE CREDITS

Photos 1–4, 6–8, 11–13, 18–21, 26, 27, 31–36, 40, 42, 44–47, 49–57, 59–66, 68, 71, and 72 by Jill Rabin

Photos 5 and 69 by Merideth Mack

Photo 9 by Yonah Sturmwind

Photos 10, 37, 43, and 70 by Chereesca Bejasa

Photo 14 by Deborah Milhaupt

Photo 15 by Megan Zintek

Photos 16 and 17 by Hollyce Hammond

Photo 22 by Shannon Korab

Photo 23 by Melanie Nadell

Photo 24 by Megan Holloway

Photo 25 by Danielle Chu

Photo 28 by Ariell Lipsky

Photo 29 by Kristen Smaldone

Photo 30 by Maria Milicevic

Photo 38 by Falon Stankowicz

Photo 39 by Sara Schoenenberger

Photo 41 by Jaime White

Photo 48 by Rachel Goode

Photo 58 by Gill Rapley

Photo 67 by Carolyn Chambers

ACKNOWLEDGMENTS

There are many people without whose help and support this book would not have been possible. Top of the list is Gail Macklin, who unwittingly set the whole thing in motion when she loaned Jill her copy of Gill's DVD back in 2010. We will be forever in her debt. Next up is Lori Overland, who was prepared to put her initial skepticism on hold and really look at the evidence Jill shared with her of how ABLW could work for babies with feeding challenges, and was then willing to share a stage with her to an audience of their peers. Thank you, Lori—it's a fantastic feeling when someone you respect steps up to show their support.

We are indebted to a number of people who offered us their professional advice and support and provided input based on their expertise: Diane Bahr, Dr. Kevin Boyd, Carrie Cicciu-Singer, Michelle Emmanuel, Catherine Watson Genna, Rachel Goode, Margot Maresky, Meghan McMillin, Agnieszka Moroni, Megan Murphy, Sara Quirk, Kary Rappaport, and Lillian

Gray Scott. Thank you; your assistance has been invaluable.

Huge thanks go to the parents who shared their stories with us, and to those who gave us permission to print photos of their babies. Practical firsthand accounts and authentic images bring the theory to life and demonstrate the difference a baby-led approach can make to babies who might otherwise struggle to assert their autonomy. We are grateful, too, to those parents and professionals who supplied us with snapshot quotes of their take on the value of ABLW. Their insightful comments enhanced our own understanding of what ABLW can offer.

We are grateful to Chereesca Bejasa, Sabrina Smiley Evans, Terri Gartenberg, PhD, Kimberly Grenawitzke, Amy Manojlovski, and Tracey Murkett for taking the time to read and give us feedback on our draft manuscript. Their comments and insights led directly to improvements in the text. Thanks are also due to our editor, Batya Rosenblum, for her patience and attention to detail.

Finally, we want to thank our long-suffering families for their tolerance and support, and for supplying us with food while we were holed up with our computers. We love you guys.

INDEX

NOTES: Page numbers followed by a *t* indicate a table; page numbers followed by an *i* indicate an illustration; page numbers followed by an *n* indicate an endnote.

The insert in the middle of the book has 72 photographs numbered in sequential order. The index refers to them as *photo xx*, where *xx* is the photo number.

ABOUT THE AUTHORS

JILL RABIN, MS, CCC-SLP/L, IBCLC, is a pediatric speech pathologist and International Board-Certified Lactation Consultant. Her areas of specialty include facilitating breast-feeding in at-risk populations, such as preterm infants with Down syndrome; using baby-led weaning and adapted baby-led weaning (ABLW) to assist babies with feeding challenges to transition to solid foods; and helping parents to implement child-directed and responsive feeding techniques in babies and children with feeding aversion. She is a respected international speaker and has been a featured guest on a number of podcasts. Jill lives in Northbrook, Illinois, with her husband. They have two grown children.

jillrabin.com | 📷 jillrabinablw

GILL RAPLEY, PhD, is known as the pioneer of baby-led weaning, having developed the theory while studying babies' developmental readiness for solids as part of her master's degree. She subsequently gained a PhD for her research comparing spoon-feeding with self-feeding. Gill has been a public health nurse, midwife, IBCLC, and voluntary breastfeeding counselor. She is the coauthor with Tracey Murkett of several books on parenting and infant feeding, including the seminal *Baby-Led Weaning: The Essential Guide*, which is now in over twenty languages. Gill lives in Kent, England, with her husband. They have three grown children and one grandchild.

ALSO IN THE BABY-LED WEANING SERIES

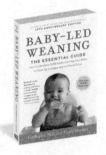

Baby-Led Weaning: The Essential Guide
How to Introduce Solid Foods and Help Your Baby
to Grow Up a Happy and Confident Eater

$16.95 US | $21.95 CAN | 256 pages
Trade paperback: 978-1-61519-558-9
Ebook: 978-1-61519-559-6

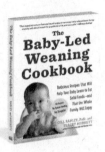

The Baby-Led Weaning Cookbook
Delicious Recipes That Will Help Your Baby
Learn to Eat Solid Foods—and That the Whole
Family Will Enjoy

$16.95 US | $21.95 CAN | 192 pages
Color illustrations throughout
Trade paperback: 978-1-61519-049-2
Ebook: 978-1-61519-168-0

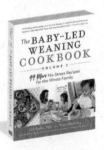

The Baby-Led Weaning Cookbook—Volume 2
99 More No-Stress Recipes for the Whole Family

$16.95 US | $21.95 CAN | 192 pages
46 color photographs
Trade paperback: 978-1-61519-621-0
Ebook: 978-1-61519-623-4

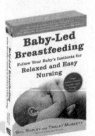

Baby-Led Breastfeeding
Follow Your Baby's Instincts for Relaxed
and Easy Nursing

$14.95 US | $22.95 CAN | 320 pages
8-page four-color photo insert
Trade paperback: 978-1-61519-066-9
Ebook: 978-1-61519-164-2